Physiology for Anaesthesiologists

T0186589

Physiology for Anaesthesiologists

Edited by

JP Howard Fee MD PhD FFARCSI
Department of Anaesthetics and Intensive Care Medicine
Queen's University of Belfast
Belfast, UK

James G Bovill MD FCARCSI FRCA
Department of Anaesthesiology
Leiden University Medical Centre
Leiden, The Netherlands

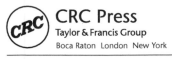
CRC Press
Taylor & Francis Group
Boca Raton London New York

CRC Press is an imprint of the
Taylor & Francis Group, an **informa** business
A TAYLOR & FRANCIS BOOK

CRC Press
Taylor & Francis Group
6000 Broken Sound Parkway NW, Suite 300
Boca Raton, FL 33487-2742

First issued in paperback 2019

ISBN-13: 978-1-84184-235-6 (hbk)
ISBN-13: 978-0-367-39376-2 (pbk)

A CIP record for this book is available from the British Library.

Library of Congress Cataloging-in-Publication Data

Data available on application

**Visit the Taylor & Francis Web site at
http://www.taylorandfrancis.com**

**and the CRC Press Web site at
http://www.crcpress.com**

Contents

Contributors

Yogen Amin
Imperial School of Anaesthesia
442 Finchley Road
London NW2 2HY
UK

Paul CM van den Berg
Intensive Care
Leiden University Medical Centre
Albinusdreef 2
PO Box 9600
2300 RC Leiden, The Netherlands

James G Bovill
Department of Anaesthesiology
Leiden University Medical Centre
Albinusdreef 2
PO Box 9600
2300 RC Leiden
The Netherlands

William I Campbell
Department of Anaesthetics
Ulster Community and Hospitals Trust
Dundonald
Belfast BT16 1RH
Northern Ireland

François Donati
Departement d'Anésthesie-Reanimation
Hopitaux de Brabois
4, rue du Morvan
54511 Vandoeuvre-Les-Nancy Cedex
France

Ilias IN Doxiadis
Department of Immunohaematology and Blood
Transfusion
Leiden University Medical Centre
Albinusdreef 2
PO Box 9600
2300 RC Leiden
The Netherlands

JP Howard Fee
Department of Anaesthetics and Intensive Care
Medicine
Queen's University
Belfast BT9 7BL
UK

Pierre Foëx
Nuffield Department of Anaesthetics
Radcliffe Infirmary
Oxford OX2 6HE
UK

Helen Higham
Nuffield Department of Anaesthetics
Radcliffe Infirmary
Oxford OX2 6HE
UK

Bart van Hoek
Department of Gastroenterology and
Hepatology, C4-P
Leiden University Medical Centre
PO Box 9600
2300 ZC Leiden
The Netherlands

CV Elzo Kraemer
Department of Intensive Care
Leiden University Medical Centre
PO Box 9600
2300 RC Leiden
The Netherlands

Cormack C McLoughlin
Department of Anaesthesia
Belfast City Hospital
Lisburn Road
Belfast BT9 7AB
UK

Claude Meistelman
Departement d'Anésthesie-Reanimation
Hopitaux de Brabois
4, rue du Morvan
54511 Vandoeuvre-Les-Nancy Cedex
France

Nollag O'Rourke
Department of Anaesthesia and Intensive Care
Medicine
University College Cork
Wilton, Cork
Ireland

George Shorten
Department of Anaesthesia and Intensive Care
Medicine
University College Cork
Wilton, Cork
Ireland

Martin Smith
Department of Neuroanaesthesia and
Neurocritical Care
The National Hospital for Neurology and
Surgery
Queen Square
London WC1N 3BG
UK

William FM Wallace
Department of Physiology
Medical Biology Centre
Queen's University Belfast
97 Lisburn Road
Belfast BT9 7BL
UK

Series Preface

Anaesthetists, uniquely, administer drugs intravenously and by inhalation that profoundly interfere with fundamental physiological functions such as breathing, cardiac output, blood pressure, the protective reflexes, and the perception of pain. The drugs used are often highly potent and potentially toxic. It is therefore entirely appropriate that anaesthetists are required to have a good working knowledge and understanding of pharmacological and physiological principles, and their application to anaesthesia and intensive care. As in other fields of medicine and biology, there have been marked advances in physiology and pharmacology in recent years, which seem to proceed at an ever-increasing pace. Much of what was considered 'state of the art' ten years ago is now regarded as commonplace; as a consequence, textbooks rapidly become outdated.

This book and its companion volume on pharmacology were conceived primarily to provide up-to-date information to trainees in anaesthesiology and related specialities preparing for postgraduate examinations in these subjects. In addition to core material for these examinations, topics not usually dealt with in textbooks for anaesthetists are also covered, since they can have at least an indirect relevance to the practising anaesthesiologist. These include antineoplastic drugs, drugs for epilepsy and psychiatric disorders in the pharmacology volume and immunology in the physiology volume. Although these drugs will seldom, if ever, be directly administered by an anaesthetist, anaesthetists do need to understand how their use by patients can impact on the conduct of anaesthesia. There is also a growing awareness of the impact of anaesthesia and surgery on the immune response, and its potential relevance for patients who have undergone, or about to undergo, organ transplantation. Alterations in the immune system can also have a direct, and sometimes dramatic effect during anaesthesia (e.g. an anaphylactic reaction to an anaesthetic drug).

While we have attempted to produce volumes that are comprehensive and clinically relevant, they are not intended to be authoritative works of reference. Thus we have been restrictive in the use of references, preferring instead to add additional reading lists, or references to recent reviews, at the end of individual chapters. We hope this will be useful for readers wishing to supplement the material covered in the volumes.

Satisfying the examiners, however, is not the end of the story. Postgraduate education is a continuing process, and we hope that this series will also be of benefit to established anaesthesiologists, and those in other related specialities, who want to keep up to date with recent developments in physiology and pharmacology.

As editors we are indebted to the individual authors for their valuable contributions to this series. We also wish to acknowledge the support of the publishers, Taylor & Francis Medical, and in particular the editorial support and encouragement provided by Maire Harris (who was very much involved in the conception of the volumes), Robert Peden and Giovanna Ceroni.

JP Howard Fee
James G Bovill

1

Cardiovascular physiology

Pierre Foëx, Helen Higham

CARDIAC MUSCLE CONTRACTION

The cardiac cell

The cardiac cells (myocytes) are branched filament-like structures 10-20 μm in diameter and 50–100 μm long. Approximately every 2 μm in their longitudinal axis, transverse (T) tubules penetrate the cells. Transmembrane calcium channels are located in the transverse tubules in the immediate vicinity of calcium release channels (ryanodine channels), which are part of the membrane of the sarcoplasmic reticulum. The close proximity of these transmembrane channels facilitates the process of excitation–contraction coupling (Figure 1.1). Ion fluxes in and out of the myocytes, the sarcoplasmic reticulum, and the mitochondria are controlled by channels and pumps in their membranes. Sodium, calcium, and potassium ion fluxes are central to the process of depolarisation (Na^+, Ca^{2+}) excitation–contraction coupling (Ca^{2+}), and repolarisation (K^+).

Within the myocytes, the basic contractile unit is the sarcomere, composed of filaments of actin and myosin. The thick filament of myosin is formed by approximately 300 individual molecules of myosin and is about 1.5 μm long and 10–15 nm wide. Each molecule possesses a bilobed head. Half of the heads are oriented towards one end of the sarcomere and half towards the other. The thin filament of actin contains two helical chains of actin supported by tropomyosin molecules with troponin complexes placed at intervals of 38 nm. Troponin C, to which calcium binds, is part of a complex that includes troponin I (the inhibitory protein for the interaction of actin and myosin) and troponin T, which links the troponin complex to tropomyosin.

Contraction of the myocytes

Following depolarisation, calcium ions enter the myocytes during the plateau phase of the action potential. This causes a triggered release of calcium through the ryanodine channels of the sarcoplasmic reticulum. The rapid increase in myoplasmic calcium results in calcium becoming available to bind with troponin C. This, in turn, removes the inhibitory effect of troponin I on the interaction of actin and myosin. Hydrolysis of adenosine triphosphate (ATP) allows the thick and thin filaments to slide past each other. The lateral projections of the myosin filaments, with their articulated heads attached to an arm that is capable of sustaining tension, give the sliding of the filaments an oar-like motion. When the arms abduct, the heads come closer to the actin filament and cross-bridges are formed at the level of active sites. Head rotation pulls on the arm and causes the actin filament to move with respect to the myosin filament (Figure 1.2). This results in both force development and shortening. The total force developed in this process is a function of the number of

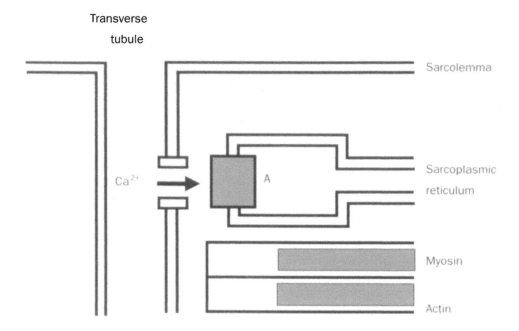

Figure 1.1 *Schematic representation of a calcium channel located in a transverse tubule in the immediate vicinity of a ryanodine receptor (A) of the sarcoplasmic reticulum.*

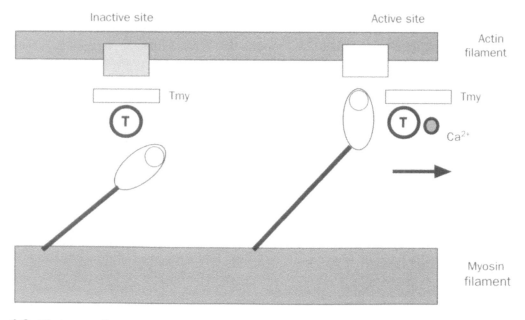

Figure 1.2 *Diagrammatic representation of actin and myosin filaments. The lateral projections of the rotating heads of myosin can attach to the actin filaments when inactive sites become active. This occurs when calcium ions become attached to tropocin (T), thus causing a change in the configuration of tropomyosin (Tmy), allowing the interaction of actin and myosin.*

cross-bridges formed. Formation of each cross-bridge requires one molecule of ATP. In addition to initiating the contractile cycle, calcium ions alter the kinetics of cross-bridge formation by altering the myosin ATPase activity: this is the fundamental mechanism of increases in the rate of cross-bridge formation, i.e. increases in contractility.

THE CARDIAC CYCLE

Each cardiac cycle consists of a period of contraction (systole) followed by a period of relaxation (diastole) (Figure 1.3). Atrial systole is initiated by the spontaneous generation of an action potential in the sino-atrial node. After a delay due to the slow conduction velocity of the atrioventricular node, the ventricles are activated and systole begins. In its early phase, the mitral, tricuspid, aortic, and pulmonary valves are closed and the ventricles contract isovolumically. Once the ventricular pressures exceed the aortic and pulmonary pressures, ejection starts. It will cease once the ventricular pressures become smaller than the aortic and pulmonary pressures. Ventricular pressures then decrease without change in volume because the atrioventricular valves are also closed: relaxation is isovolumic. Once the ventricular pressures are smaller than the atrial pressures, the atrioventricular valves open and filling starts. Note that ventricular emptying and ventricular filling are fastest at the beginning of ejection and filling respectively.

Ventricular filling, after its early rapid phase, becomes much slower or even stops (diastasis), until it is completed by atrial contraction. Opening and, respectively, closure of the aortic and pulmonary valves are responsible for the first and second heart sounds.

For each cardiac cycle, the instantaneous relationship between ventricular pressure and volume forms a pressure–volume loop. The loop has four segments representing isovolumic contraction, ejection, isovolumic relaxation, and filling. The width of the loop represents the stroke volume; its surface area represents the stroke work. For a given ventricle and for a constant inotropic state, the loops are bounded by the

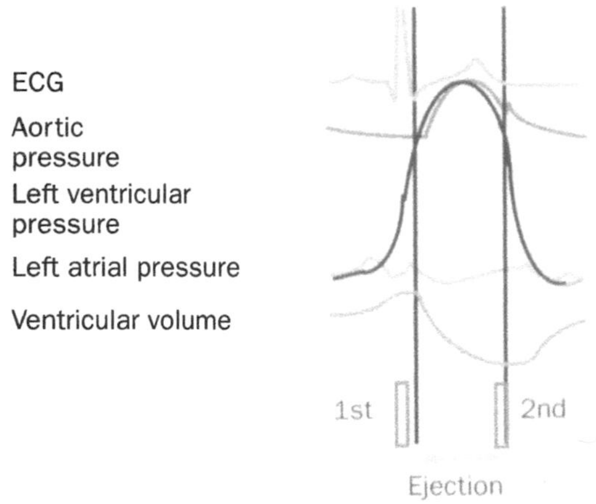

ECG
Aortic pressure
Left ventricular pressure
Left atrial pressure
Ventricular volume

1st   2nd

Ejection

Figure 1.3 *Various waveforms that characterise the cardiac cycle: electrocardiogram (ECG), aortic pressure, left ventricular pressure, left atrial pressure, and left ventricular volume, with schematic representation of the first and second heart sounds.*

end-diastolic pressure–volume relationship (an expression of ventricular stiffness), and the end-systolic pressure–volume relationship, which represents the contractile state of the myocardium. Positive inotropic interventions increase, while negative inotropy decreases the slope of the end-systolic pressure–volume relationship, also termed the maximum elastance.

REGULATION OF CARDIAC FUNCTION

Performance of the heart as a muscle and as a pump is influenced by three major determinants: resistance to contraction/ejection (the afterload), initial fibre length/ventricular filling (the preload), and changes in the contractile state of the cardiac muscle (contractility, inotropy). In the face of ventricular hypertrophy and/or ischaemia, ventricular compliance (or its inverse, ventricular stiffness) becomes an important determinant of pump function.

Preload

The resting length of the sarcomeres is the true preload of the cardiac muscle: its relationship to the force developed during contraction is the cellular basis of Starling's law of the heart. Maximum force can be developed when the resting sarcomere length is 2.2 μm. At greater sarcomere lengths, the scope for cross-bridge formation is reduced because the actin and myosin filaments are too far apart. At smaller sarcomere lengths, the filaments are farther apart rather than buckled; this reduces the number of cross-bridges that can be formed.

In the intact heart, the end-diastolic pressure of the ventricles is commonly used as representing the preload. For the left ventricle, the pulmonary artery occluded pressure (pulmonary wedge pressure) is generally used to represent the preload. Changes in preload are associated with changes in stroke volume, stroke work, and cardiac output. The relationship between cardiac output and end-diastolic pressure is curvilinear (ventricular function curve). This is the expression of Starling's law of the heart (Figure 1.4).

Contractility

In the isolated heart muscle and in the intact heart, for a given preload, force development and stroke volume can be increased by positive or decreased by negative inotropic interventions, resulting in upwards or downwards shifts of the ventricular function curve (Figure 1.4).

Changes in the inotropic state of the myocardium ultimately result from either an increase in myoplasmic calcium or increased sensitivity of the contractile apparatus to calcium. Increases in myoplasmic calcium result from receptor-mediated increases in cyclic adenosine monophosphate (cAMP) (β-adrenoceptor stimulation) or reduced breakdown of cAMP (phosphodiesterase inhibitors).

Increased sensitivity to calcium is an important factor in the preload dependence of force development, suggesting that the degree of actin–myosin overlap may not be the critical factor in Starling's law of the heart. Thus the effects of preload and contractility on cardiac muscle performance may relate to the same mechanism, i.e. a reduced inhibition of actin–myosin interaction due to changes in troponin I.

CONTROL OF CARDIAC OUTPUT

Cardiac output (the product of heart rate and stroke volume) averages 5.0 l/min in a resting 70 kg supine man. It can increase fivefold with strenuous exercise. Variations in cardiac output can be produced by changes in heart rate or stroke volume. Heart rate is controlled primarily by the autonomic nervous system: sympathetic stimulation increases while parasympathetic stimulation decreases the cardiac rate. The stroke volume is determined by three main factors: preload, afterload, and contractility. Preload and afterload are highly sensitive to changes in metabolic requirements (whole-body oxygen consumption). Where local regulation causes peripheral or splanchnic vasodilatation, venous return is increased so that the preload of the ventricles is augmented; at the same time, resistance to left ventricular ejection is reduced, allowing stroke volume to increase. Preload, afterload, and contractility are influenced by the autonomic nervous system. α Adrenergic stimulation causes arteriolar and venoconstriction. β Adrenoceptor stimulation increases contractility. Parasympathetic stimulation decreases vascular resistance and depresses cardiac contractility.

RHYTHMICITY OF THE HEART

Cardiac cells that are capable of developing spontaneous diastolic depolarisation are called pacemaker cells; they generate the cardiac rhythm. Normally, the dominant pacemaker of the heart is the sinus node. In adults, it fires at a rate of 60–100 beats/min. Cells capable of developing spontaneous diastolic depolarisation are also found in specialised fibres in the atria, the atrioventricular node, and the His–Purkinje system. These cells exhibit a slower rate of spontaneous depolarisation than the sinus node.

Spontaneous depolarisation of pacemaker cells results from ionic currents across the cell membrane, including a non-specific inward current followed by a transient inward calcium current carried by T-type calcium channels. Depolarisation spreads from the sino-atrial node to the atrial tissue, initiating atrial contraction, and towards the atrioventricular node where

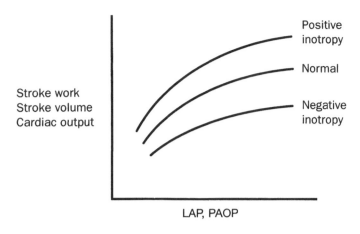

Figure 1.4 *Left ventricular function curves demonstrating the upward and downward shifts caused by an increase, respectively decrease, of contractility. LAP, left atrial pressure; PAOP, pulmonary capillary wedge pressure.*

conduction is slow so that activation of the ventricles through the bundle of this is delayed, allowing atria to contribute to ventricular filling before ventricular contraction starts.

The action potential consists of a transient, local trans-sarcolemmal depolarising current that raises the transmembrane potential from its resting value (-80 to –90 mV) to a slightly positive value (Figure 1.5). In contractile cells, the earliest and largest component of membrane depolarisation is the rapid inward influx of sodium ions. The resting potential is established and maintained by the trans-sarcolemmal Na^+/K^+-ATPase that pumps sodium ions out of the cytoplasm.

In contractile cells, calcium influx through more slowly opening channels produces the plateau phase of the action potential, while potassium efflux through two types of potassium channels produces both the inward rectifier current (I_{KI}) and the delayed rectifier current (I_K). By contrast, in rhythmically discharging cells (pacemaker cells), the resting membrane potential declines to the threshold level at which depolarisation, carried largely by calcium ions, occurs. Spontaneous depolarisation is due to calcium entry through T-type channels, while acute depolarisation is due to calcium entry through L-type channels. At the peak of depolarisation, potassium channels open and repolarisation is initiated, so there is no plateau phase (Figure 1.5).

Control of heart rate by the autonomic nervous system results from changes in the speed of spontaneous depolarisation. Vagal stimulation hyperpolarises the cell membrane and increases the potassium conductance of nodal tissue via M_2 muscarinic receptors, G protein, and special potassium channels. As a result, the decay of the inward rectifier current (I_K) is reduced. Simulation of M_2 muscarinic receptors also decreases cAMP in the cells. This in turn slows the opening of calcium channels so that spontaneous depolarisation is further reduced, leading to vagally mediated bradycardia.

With sympathetic stimulation, activation of β-adrenoceptors increases cAMP, facilitating the opening of T-type calcium channels so that spontaneous depolarisation is facilitated, even though the cell membrane is hyperpolarised.

THE ELECTROCARDIOGRAM

As the body is a volume conductor, the action potentials of myocardial fibres can be recorded at the body surface, where their algebraic sum is recorded as the electrocardiogram (ECG) (Figure 1.6).

The ECG may be recorded by an active electrode connected to an indifferent electrode (zero potential) or by two active electrodes (unipolar and bipolar leads respectively). The six conventional leads are unipolar. The sequence in which different parts of the heart are depolarised and the position of the heart with respect to the electrodes determine the configuration of the waves recorded by each lead. Because of the timing and direction of propagation of the

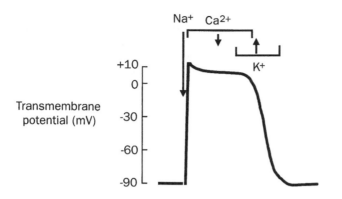

Figure 1.5 *Schematic representation of the three major ion fluxes that are responsible for the action potential of contractile cardiac cells.*

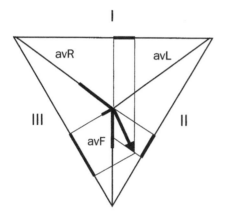

Figure 1.6 *Diagrammatic representation of the six standard leads of the ECG. The arrow represents the vector of cardiac activation and the thick lines represent its projection on the six leads.*

depolarisation, the normal ECG waveform does not exhibit the plateau phase seen at cellular level.

Arrhythmias

In the normal heart, each beat originates in the sino-atrial node. Heart rate in young individuals varies with respiration, accelerating during inspiration and slowing during expiration: sinus arrhythmia is a normal phenomenon and is due primarily to fluctuations in parasympathetic outflow to the heart. Disease processes affecting the sinus node may lead to profound bradycardia.

Altered normal automaticity refers to a change in the rate of pacemaker discharge caused by loss of 'overdrive suppression' by the sino-atrial node or loss of electrotonic depression by adjacent fibres. Latent pacemakers are then able to take over from the normal pacemaker.

Abnormal automaticity results from altered ionic fluxes and occurs in fibres that do not normally exhibit automaticity, i.e. atrial or ventricular contractile fibres. Afterdepolarisations are oscillations in the transmembrane potential that follow the upstroke of the action potential. These may trigger sustained rhythmic activity. Early afterdepolarisations occur before, and delayed afterdepolarisations after, the full repolarisation phase of the action potential. Delayed afterdepolarisations usually result from calcium overload, which may in turn be caused by triggered calcium release. Digitalis excess is a cause of delayed afterdepolarisations; catecholamines and myocardial ischaemia also facilitate delayed afterdepolarisations resulting in triggered rhythmic activity.

Re-entry of excitation is another major mechanism of arrhythmias. The propagating action potentials normally die out following sequential activation of atrial or ventricular tissue. Under abnormal circumstances, the propagating action potentials do not die out but persist and re-excite non-refractory tissue, giving rise to extrasystole, or tachycardia. In order for re-entry excitation to occur, an area of unidirectional conduction block and a re-entrant pathway allowing excitation to return to its point of origin are necessary (Figure 1.7). Sino-atrial and atrioventricular nodes, because of their relatively slow conduction velocity and prolonged refractoriness, are preferential sites for re-entry. Re-entry in the atrioventricular node occurs when an accessory pathway is present, so that conduction is fast in one pathway and slow in the other.

Altered automaticity is responsible for sinus bradycardia, sinus tachycardia, sinus arrhythmia, atrioventricular junctional rhythm, idioventricular rhythm, and wandering atrial pacemaker.

Abnormal automaticity results in slow monomorphic ventricular tachycardia, some ectopic atrial tachycardia, accelerated atrioventricular rhythm, and accelerated idioventricular rhythm.

Triggered rhythmic activity is responsible for reperfusion ventricular tachycardia, catecholamine-induced ventricular tachycardia, ectopic atrial tachycardia, and polymorphic ventricular tachycardia.

Re-entrant excitation causes atrial flutter, atrial fibrillation, atrioventricular reciprocating tachycardia (Wolff–Parkinson–White, Lown–Ganong–Levine syndromes), paroxysmal supraventricular tachycardia, and some ventricular tachycardia associated with myocardial ischaemia.

NEUROHUMORAL CONTROL OF THE CIRCULATION

Cardiovascular regulation needs to maintain a relatively constant arterial pressure and to provide sufficient perfusion to meet metabolic demands. Neurohumoral control of arterial pressure is mediated through changes in cardiac output and/or peripheral vascular resistance. Acute mechanisms for blood pressure regulation are coordinated in the brainstem in the cardiovascular control centres (Figure 1.8). These are influenced by impulses from other neural centres and by sensors in the circulation. Endogenous mediators released into the bloodstream contribute to the regulation of the circulation. The centres for cardiovascular control are located in the medulla oblongata and lower pons, close to the centres regulating respiration.

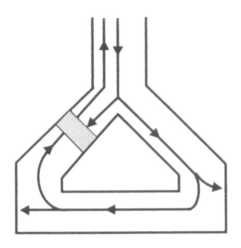

Figure 1.7 Schematic representation of re-entry, one of the frequent cause of dysrhythmias. The hatched zone represents unidirectional block (anterograde), which allows retrograde progression of impulses, leading to further activation.

Neural control

The centres for circulatory control include two divisions – vasomotor and cardiac – which supply the peripheral vasculature and the heart respectively. The vasomotor centre in turn has a vasoconstrictor area, termed C-1, containing a high density of noradrenaline-secreting neurones; it has also a vasodilator region, termed A-1. This region inhibits the activity of the vasoconstrictor region. C-1 neurones synapse with cells in the intermediolateral cell column, which synapse further with adrenergic neurones. The adrenergic neurones send vasoconstrictor fibres to the periphery.

The cardiac control centre is subdivided into cardio-inhibitory and cardiostimulatory areas. The nucleus ambiguus and the dorsal nucleus of the vagus nerve are cardio-inhibitory via the parasympathetic system. Areas of the lateral medulla act as cardiostimulatory centres via the sympathetic nervous system. Both regions are tonically active, and the proximity of the cardiostimulator and vasomotor areas is responsible for the basal arteriolar tone. The control

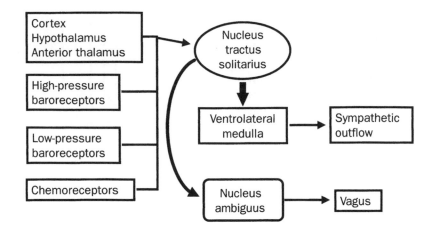

Figure 1.8 *Diagrammatic representation of the central control of the circulation, showing the influence of higher centres and of baro- and chemoreceptors on the cardiovascular centre.*

centres receive inputs from other regions: the reticular substance of the pons, mesencephalon, diencephalon, hypothalamus, and many other areas, including the motor cortex.

The autonomic nervous system provides innervation to the heart and the peripheral circulation. The sympathetic and parasympathetic systems are physiologically antagonistic (Table 1.1). The effects on the heart of sympathetic stimulation include tachycardia, increased conduction velocity, increased automaticity, and increased contractility. The effects on the vasculature differ. Sympathetic stimulation constricts skin and mucosal vessels, while in skeletal muscles constriction is via α_1 receptors and dilation is via β_2 receptors. Similarly, the coronary circulation exhibits α_1 adrenoceptor-mediated vasoconstriction and β_2 adrenoceptor-mediated vasodilatation. Sympathetic stimulation causes pulmonary vasoconstriction. Parasympathetic stimulation has essentially opposite effects, i.e. it causes bradycardia and decreases conduction, with little effect on contractility. Parasympathetic stimulation causes peripheral vasodilation. However, as vasodilatation is mediated by the endothelium (release of nitric oxide, NO), vasoconstriction (mediated by muscarinic receptors) occurs when the endothelium is damaged, as this prevents the release of NO.

Humoral control of the circulation

Catecholamines are released by the adrenal medulla, which is innervated by preganglionic sympathetic fibres. The adrenal medulla secretes mostly adrenaline (80%). Adrenaline and noradrenaline released in the bloodstream function as hormones. Their effects on the heart and the circulation are similar to those of sympathetic stimulation.

The renin–angiotensin–aldosterone system is another humoral regulator of the cardiovascular system (Figure 1.9). The juxtaglomerular cells of the renal cortex synthesise and release the enzyme renin. The cells are located close to the afferent arterioles of the glomeruli. The secretion of renin is stimulated by a decrease in renal artery pressure, reduced sodium delivery to the distal tubule, and sympathetic stimulation (activation of β_1 adrenoceptors). Renin cleaves angiotensinogen to form a decapeptide: angiotensin I. The latter is inactive but is hydrolysed by angiotensin-converting enzyme (ACE) into an active octapeptide: angiotensin II. This conversion takes place predominantly in the vascular endothelium of the lungs. Angiotensin II is a powerful vasoconstrictor. It also stimulates transmission in the sympathetic nervous system and increases the release of noradrenaline via

Table 1.1 Effects of sympathetic and parasympathetic stimulation on the heart and the circulation

	Sympathetic stimulation	Parasympathetic stimulation
Heart		
Heart rate	Increased	Decreased
Contractility	Increased	Decreased
Conduction	Increased	Decreased
Splanchnic vessels	Constricted	
Coronary arteries		
Direct effect	Constricted	Dilated
Demand-mediated effect	Dilated	Constricted

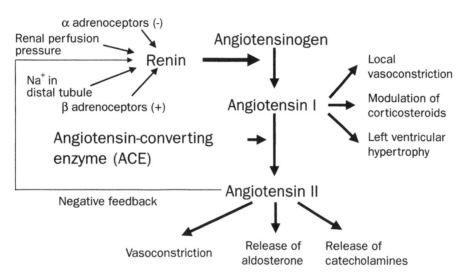

Figure 1.9 *The renin–angiotensin–aldosterone system is central to the long-term control of blood pressure and, via angiotensin II, to the short-term control of vasomotor tone.*

activation of presynaptic angiotensin II receptors. By direct stimulation of the adrenal cortex, angiotensin II increases the synthesis and secretion of aldosterone. Aldosterone causes sodium and water retention, leading to expansion of the plasma volume: this facilitates an increase in arterial pressure. Angiotensin II is metabolised by aminopeptidases into inactive metabolites and an active heptapeptide: angiotensin III, which is a potent stimulant of aldosterone.

Haemorrhage and dehydration reduce arterial pressure and sodium delivery to the macula densa. This increases the release of renin, and therefore promotes the formation of angiotensins II and III.

Vasopressin, or antidiuretic hormone, is synthesised in the supraoptic and paraventricular nuclei of the brainstem and is transported to the posterior pituitary gland. Its release occurs in response to an increase in plasma osmolality (sensed by the hypothalamic osmoreceptors), a decrease in plasma volume (sensed mostly by atrial receptors), or an increase in plasma concentration of angiotensin II. Vasopressin increases water reabsorption in the collecting ducts of the kidney by stimulating vasopressin receptors. In addition, vasopressin is a powerful vasoconstrictor, especially in the skin and the gastrointestinal tract, although coronary arteries are also constricted.

Atrial natriuretic peptide (ANP) is synthesised and stored in atrial myocytes: distension of the atria, especially the right atrium, causes the release of ANP, which relaxes vascular smooth muscle, decreases sympathetic tone, and promotes natriuresis and glomerular filtration. ANP also suppresses vasopressin secretion.

Nitric oxide is an important cell messenger. It relaxes vascular smooth muscle via the activation of soluble guanylyl cyclase, leading to the formation of cyclic guanosine monophosphate (cGMP). In turn, cGMP activates a protein kinase such that calcium is extruded from the cell via activation of a calcium ATPase.

Reflex control of the circulation

Arterial (high-pressure) baroreceptors are present in the aortic arch and internal carotid arteries (carotid sinus). Afferent fibres travel in the aortic and carotid sinus nerves, which, via the vagus and glossopharyngeal nerves, connect with the cardiovascular centres. When the baroreceptor endings are stretched, tonic nerve discharge increases in proportion to the pressure change in the baroreceptors. These afferent inputs increase the activity of the medullary depressor area so that pressor and cardiac areas are inhibited, causing bradycardia and reducing both contractility and vasomotor tone. The baroreceptor reflex is a major contributor to the rapid control of blood pressure, especially during changes in posture. The response is greatest over the physiological range (80–150 mmHg) and is more accentuated for reductions than for increases in blood pressure. The sensitivity of the baroreflex can be tested by the administration of a vasodilator (sodium nitroprusside) or a vasoconstrictor (phenylephrine). The slope of the relationship between the R–R interval of the ECG and arterial pressure indicates the sensitivity of the baroreflex. The baroreceptors adapt to prolonged changes in arterial pressure. In hypertensive patients, the baroreflex is reset at higher levels.

Atrial and venous low-pressure baroreceptors are localised near the junction of the superior and inferior venae cavae with the right atrium. They respond to increases in central venous pressure. They send impulses through myelinated fibres of the vagus nerves to the central nervous system. The afferent impulses travel in the sympathetic fibres to the sino-atrial node. The tachycardia in response to atrial distension constitutes the Bainbridge reflex. Like the arterial baroreceptors, the atrial receptors adapt to a continuous increase in atrial pressure.

The ventricles contain receptors sensitive to stretch and to strong contractions. Inputs travel to the medulla via unmyelinated vagal fibres and elicit a decrease in sympathetic tone, causing bradycardia and vasodilatation.

While the arterial chemoreceptors predominantly cause an increase in ventilation, their secondary effect is to produce sympathetic vasoconstriction during hypotension, in addition to that caused by arterial baroreceptors.

The overall function of the baroreceptors can be tested by monitoring the changes in pressure and heart rate that occur during a short period of straining: the Valsalva manoeuvre. By forcing expiration against a closed glottis, there is an initial increase in blood pressure caused by the increase in intrathoracic pressure (Figure 1.10). Pressure then falls because the increase in intrathoracic pressure has reduced venous return and cardiac output. This fall in pressure, via the baroreceptors, causes tachycardia and an increase in peripheral vascular resistance. When intrathoracic pressure is allowed to return to normal on opening the glottis, cardiac output is restored but, as the peripheral vascular resistance is still elevated, blood pressure rises above normal. This stimulates the baroreceptor so that bradycardia and a reduction in vascular resistance will follow. In patients with widespread autonomic dysfunction, the heart-rate changes are absent.

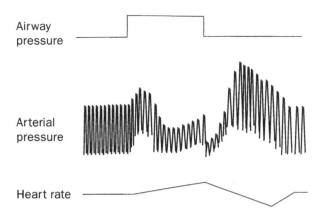

Airway
pressure

Arterial
pressure

Heart rate

Figure 1.10 *Schematic representation of the effect of a sudden large increase in airway pressure (Valsalva manoeuvre). After an initial, short-lived increase in pressure at the beginning of the manoeuvre, reflecting the squeezing of some of the pulmonary blood volume into the left atrium, blood pressure falls. A slight increase in the later phase represents peripheral vasocontriction. At the end of the manoeuvre, there is a reduction of blood pressure due to an increase in intrapulmonary blood volume, followed by an overshoot when cardiac output is restored while vascular resistance is still increased.*

EFFECTS OF EXERCISE ON THE CIRCULATION

Blood flow in rhythmically contracting muscle increases as much as 30-fold. Local mechanisms, including a fall in tissue P_{O_2}, a rise in P_{CO_2}, and accumulation of K^+, contribute to the maintenance of high blood flow. Further dilatation results from the increase in temperature in contracting muscle. The number of open capillaries is increased 10- to 100-fold such that the diffusion distance is greatly decreased, facilitating oxygen and nutrient delivery.

Isometric exercise causes an increase in heart rate, largely due to decreased vagal tone. Within a few seconds, there is a sharp increase in systolic and diastolic blood pressure but little change in stroke volume. The response to isotonic exercise is also characterised by a prompt

increase in heart rate; this is associated with a marked increase in stroke volume. In addition, peripheral vascular resistance decreases. As a consequence, systolic blood pressure rises moderately and diastolic pressure remains unchanged or falls. Cardiac output may increase to 35 l/min as a result of increased heart rate and stroke volume, the latter being facilitated by increased contractility. These changes result from increased sympathetic and decreased parasympathetic discharge. Venous return is increased by mobilisation of blood from the splanchnic circulation.

EFFECTS OF HAEMORRHAGE

Haemorrhage decreases venous return, so that cardiac output falls. The arterial baroreceptors are stretched to a lesser degree, so that sympathetic output is increased. This results in an increase in heart rate and peripheral vasoconstriction. The latter is generalised and spares only the cerebral and, to an extent, coronary circulations. In the brain, the vasoconstrictor innervation is insignificant, while in the coronary circulation, flow is still increased because of the tachycardia. The reflex venoconstriction of the splanchnic area shifts blood into the systemic circulation. This may include a small contribution from the spleen. Renal vasoconstriction occurs in both afferent and efferent arterioles, and the glomerular filtration rate is reduced. Severe hypotension causes tubular damage, including tubular necrosis.

Haemorrhage stimulates adrenal medullary secretion. However, the effects of circulating catecholamines contribute little to the vasoconstriction caused by the sympathetic nervous system. Haemorrhage also causes an increase in the level of circulating angiotensin II mediated by an increased renin release.

As the arterioles constrict, and the venous pressure falls, there is a drop in capillary pressure. This allows fluid to move from the interstitial space into the intravascular space, thus helping to restore the circulating volume. In turn, the reduction of the interstitial fluid volume causes a shift of fluid from the cells. As a result, after moderate haemorrhage, the plasma volume is restored in 12–92 hours, but red cell mass is restored much later under the control of erythropoietin.

PERIPHERAL CIRCULATION

The primary function of the microcirculation is the delivery of oxygen and fuels to the tissues as well as the removal of carbon dioxide and tissue metabolites, including hormones and metabolic mediators. Capillaries and probably smaller arterioles and venules are the main sites for gas exchange. Both the number of open capillaries and the distribution of blood within the vessels can be regulated by the precapillary sphincters. The systemic and pulmonary circulations consist of series-coupled sections.

The capillary exchange vessels are limited by a single layer of endothelial cells. They form a dense network with a large cross-sectional area, a large surface area, and a short length. Systemic capillaries have an average radius of 3 μm, a length of 750 μm, a cross-sectional area of 30 μm², and a surface area of 15 000 μm². Under resting conditions, 25–35% of the capillaries are open and their effective exchange surface is 250–350 m². The pulmonary capillaries are wider (4 μm) and shorter (350 μm) than the systemic capillaries; their effective surface area is approximately 60 m², increasing to 90 m² with heavy exercise. The average transit time through lung capillaries is about 1 s, decreasing to 0.35 s with heavy exercise.

At the capillary level, the transcapillary exchange of fluids depends upon the hydrostatic pressure in the capillaries and the colloid–osmotic pressure of the blood (Starling's hypothesis). The net rate and direction of fluid movement J_v is a function of the net filtration pressure $P_{capillary} - P_{interstitium}$ and the net colloid–osmotic pressure $\Pi_{plasma} - \Pi_{interstitium}$ corrected for the characteristics of the capillary membrane expressed as the reflection coefficient σ. In addition, filtration depends upon the surface area S and the hydraulic conductance of the wall L_p. Thus, capillary fluid exchange can be expressed as follows:

$$J_v = L_p S \left[(P_{cap.} - P_{interst.}) - \sigma (\Pi_{plasma} - \Pi_{interst.}) \right]$$

cap. = capillary; interst. = interstitium

For filtration to remain within acceptable limits, the pressure at the arteriolar end of the capillary segment considered must be about 4 kPa (30 mmHg) and the venous pressure about 2 kPa (15 mmHg). Exceptions are the glomerular capillaries of the kidneys, where the inflow pressure is of the order of 9 kPa (70 mmHg), thus ensuring net filtration. Conversely, in the lungs, the inflow pressure is normally only 1.3 kPa (10 mmHg), such that filtration is minimal. The plasma–colloid osmotic pressure, due mostly to albumin, is approximately 3 kPa (25 mmHg), thus ensuring that in the lungs and in most capillary beds, net filtration is limited. The equilibrium of hydrostatic and colloid–osmotic forces can be disrupted when mediators such as bradykinin, kallidin, and histamine increase capillary permeability and allow proteins to leak into the interstitial space. Tissue oedema may result from excessive hydrostatic pressure, reduced colloid–osmotic pressure, increased permeability, or obstruction of lymphatic drainage. The latter is necessary in all tissues because there is always some net filtration into the interstitial space.

For uncharged soluble particles, diffusion depends upon the diffusion constant and the concentration difference per unit distance. Lipid-soluble substances diffuse almost freely whereas water-soluble substances pass slowly through the endothelial cells. However, for small water-soluble molecules, smaller than the endothelial pore size, diffusion is free – but only across the pore area. For large molecules, diffusion is very restricted and additional diffusion is only possible through large pores or capillary leaks.

The capillary bed is controlled by the characteristics of the pre- and postcapillary resistance vessels. The precapillary resistance vessels (small arteries and arterioles) offer the larger part of the total resistance to blood flow. Small changes in their radius cause large changes in resistance. While at each branching, the combined cross-sectional area of the branches exceeds that of the stem, the radius of each branch is smaller than that of the stem. As resistance varies as the fourth power of the radius, resistance increases with each branching. Besides offering a high resistance to blood inflow into the capillaries, thus protecting them against excessive hydraulic pressure, the pre-capillary sphincters determine the size of the capillary exchange area by altering the number of open capillaries.

The postcapillary resistance vessels (venules and small veins) determine the ratio between pre- and postcapillary resistance. This controls the hydrostatic pressure in the capillaries and therefore contributes to the regulation of fluid transfer. The large cross-sectional area, large volume, and low resistance of the postcapillary resistance vessels allow venous return along a low pressure gradient.

Veins have a small amount of elastin and smooth muscle in their walls. Pressure at the end of capillaries is approximately 1.3 kPa (10 mmHg) and at the entrance of the vena cava in the heart approximately 0.5 kPa (4 mmHg). The venous system contains about two-thirds of the total blood volume, and may take up to 90% of fluid loads.

By contrast with veins, arteries contain an internal elastic membrane in their media. This allows the systolic storage of blood and its diastolic propulsion between cardiac contractions. Large arteries offer little resistance to flow and, as they are distensible, damp the pulsatile output of the ventricles. When blood reaches the smaller arteries of the systemic circulation, flow is relatively steady. By contrast, flow remains pulsatile throughout the pulmonary circulation.

As arteries subdivide, the proportion of elastic fibres decreases and the walls become thinner so that in arterioles the media consist almost entirely of smooth muscle with a rich nerve supply. The ability to regulate arteriolar calibre is central to the distribution of blood flow to meet local metabolic requirements. In addition, changes of arteriolar calibre are fundamental to the maintenance of arterial pressure in the face of changing cardiac output.

Resistance in the circulation

In pure hydraulic systems, the pressure difference $(P_1 - P_2)$ across a tube and its resistance R to flow determine the flow Q as

$$Q = \frac{P_1 - P_2}{R}$$

The resistance depends upon the viscosity η of the fluid, the length L of the tube, and its radius r:

$$R = \frac{8\eta L}{\pi r^4}$$

Poiseuille's law combines these relationships such that

$$Q = \frac{(P_1 - P_2)\,\pi r^4}{8\eta L}$$

This shows that flow depends upon the cross-sectional area of the tube (πr^2) and the velocity of the fluid, which is proportional to the square of the radius.

These relationships are often used to calculate systemic and pulmonary vascular resistances:

$$SVR = \frac{MAP - CVP}{CO}$$

and

$$PVR = \frac{MPAP - LAP}{CO}$$

where MAP is the mean arterial pressure, CVP the central venous pressure, MPAP the mean pulmonary artery pressure, LAP the left atrial pressure, and CO the cardiac output. Units for these haemodynamic variables are given in Table 1.2.

Viscosity η is one of the determinants of vascular resistance, it is the resistance to flow due to the friction of molecules in the moving stream. It depends mainly on the concentration of the

Table 1.2 Normal values and units of haemodynamic variables

Arterial blood pressure	BP	
Systolic	SAP	90–140 mmHg
Diastolic	DAP	60–90 mmHg
Mean	MAP	70–105 mmHg
Right atrial pressure	RAP	2–6 mmHg
Right ventricular pressure	RVP	
Systolic	RVSP	15–25 mmHg
Diastolic	RVDP	0–8 mmHg
Pulmonary artery pressure	PAP	
Systolic	SPAP	15–25 mmHg
Diastolic	DPAP	8–15 mmHg
Mean	MPAP	10–20 mmHg
Pulmonary occluded pressure (pulmonary wedge pressure)	PAOP (PAWP)	6–12 mmHg
Left atrial pressure	LAP	6–12 mmHg
Cardiac output	CO	4–8 l min^{-1}
Cardiac index	CI	2.5–4.0 l min^{-1} m^{-2}
Stroke volume	SV	60–100 ml beat^{-1}
Stroke volume index	SVI	33–47 ml beat^{-1} m^{-2}
Systemic vascular resistance	SVR	800–1500 dyn s cm^{-5}
Systemic vascular resistance index	SVRI	1970–2390 dyn s cm^{-5} m^{-2}
Pulmonary vascular resistance	PVR	<250 dyn s cm^{-5}
Pulmonary vascular resistance index	PVRI	255–285 dyn s cm^{-5} m^{-2}
Left ventricular stroke work	LVSV	58–107 g m beat^{-1}
Left ventricular stroke work index	LVSVI	37–62 g m m^{-2} beat^{-1}
Right ventricular stroke work	RVSV	8–16 g m beat^{-1}
Right ventricular stroke work index	RVSVI	5–10 g m m^{-2} beat^{-1}

red cells. Blood viscosity in vivo is less than in vitro because of axial streaming of the cells. Blood viscosity at normal haematocrit is approximately 3.6, using water as reference. With a haematocrit of 60%, it reaches 5.6.

While resistance is often calculated and used to describe the vascular beds, it is purely the static relationship between mean pressure and mean flow; the dynamic relationship between pulsatile pressure and flow (input impedance) is more meaningful because of the pulsatile nature of the circulation. This is especially true of the pulmonary circulation, where input impedance is much higher than the calculated 'static' resistance. The analogy with AC current is more appropriate than with DC current.

Control of the microcirculation

Vascular smooth muscle tone is influenced by

remote, centrally mediated, and local control mechanisms. The remote mechanisms include neural and hormonal factors.

Arteries and arterioles are innervated by sympathetic fibres. The extent of innervation varies from tissue to tissue: renal and splanchnic vessels are richly innervated while cerebral and coronary vessels are much more sparsely innervated. Neuronal supply is more abundant in larger than in smaller vessels. α adrenoceptor stimulation causes vasoconstriction, while β_2 adrenoceptor stimulation causes vasodilatation.

Many endogenously produced mediators constrict or dilate vascular smooth muscle. Adrenaline, noradrenaline, angiotensin II, vasopressin, endothelins, prostaglandin $F_{2\alpha}$ ($PGF_{2\alpha}$), and thromboxane cause vasoconstriction, while acetylcholine, atrial natriuretic peptide, bradykinin, serotonin, adenosine, and prostacyclin (PGI_2), as well as prostaglandin E_2 (PGE_2) cause vasodilatation. Many of these substances are synthesised and/or released by the endothelium in the vicinity of vascular smooth muscle and play a role in the local control of blood flow. Nitric oxide (NO) is central to the regulation of the microcirculation. This is made obvious by the large changes in systemic vascular resistance brought about by blockade of NO by the inhibitor L-NMMA (N-monomethyl-L-arginine). The magnitude of the changes in resistance, and their variability among tissues indicate that NO plays an important role in the control of blood flow.

CHARACTERISTICS OF SPECIAL CIRCULATIONS

Pulmonary circulation

The pulmonary circulation is able to accommodate the whole of the cardiac output both at rest and during maximal exercise while maintaining a low pressure so that leakage of fluid into the alveoli is prevented. This is achieved by an extremely dense capillary network, able to be recruited as a function of the demands imposed by the systemic circulation.

The 17 successive orders of branches leading to the pulmonary capillaries are short. The capillaries themselves have a diameter of 7–9 μm and a length of 9–13 μm. The number of capillary segments can be estimated to between 280 and 300×10^{-9}. Each of the 300×10^6 alveoli is in contact with 1800–2000 capillary segments. The high number of capillaries suggests that around the alveoli there is a sheet of flowing blood. The volume of blood in the pulmonary vasculature from the pulmonary valve to the alveoli is about 150 ml, while the volume in the whole of the pulmonary vascular bed is approximately 450 ml.

The resistance or, better, input impedance of the pulmonary circulation is low compared with that of the systemic circulation, and can be reduced by recruitment and distension. Recruitment means that some vessels that are closed (or open without blood flow) start to conduct blood. This mechanism is particularly important in the upper and mid zones of the lungs. Distension means that the thin-walled vessels that are already open can distend further when pressure increases. This plays an important role in the regulation of resistance in the lower zones of the lungs.

Regional differences in regulation of resistance/input impedance are associated with differences in blood flow, ventilation, gas exchange, alveolar space, and intrapleural pressure due to gravity (Figure 1.11). In the upper third of the lung, in an erect subject, the hydrostatic pressure in the pulmonary capillaries is lower than the airway pressure, and flow may be interrupted. In the middle zones, the inflow pressure is higher than the airway pressure, but the venous pressure may be lower than the airway pressure. By contrast, in the lower zone, both inflow and outflow pressures are higher than airway pressure, and flow is never interrupted. The effect of gravity is such that most of the blood flow goes to the lowermost region of the lungs.

The gravity-dependent distribution of blood flow is matched by a gravity-dependent distribution of ventilation. As the alveoli in the lower zones of the lungs are relatively compressed by the weight of the lungs, they are poorly expanded,

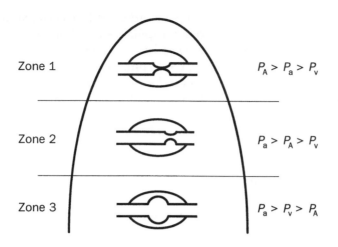

Zone 1 $P_A > P_a > P_v$

Zone 2 $P_a > P_A > P_v$

Zone 3 $P_a > P_v > P_A$

Figure 1.11 *Blood flow in the lungs is not uniform. West has defined three zones. In the uppermost lung (zone 1), alveolar pressure P_A may exceed pulmonary arterial pressure P_a such that there is little or no blood flow at times. Conversely, in the lowermost zone (zone 3), pulmonary arterial and even pulmonary venous pressure always exceed pulmonary alveolar pressure; there is always flow. This situation results from the vertical hydrostatic pressure gradient imposed by gravity.*

and therefore are more compliant than well-expanded alveoli in the upper zones of the lungs. As a result, ventilation is greater in the lower than in the upper zone of the lungs. This minimises the inequality of ventilation and perfusion and narrows the distribution of $\dot{V}/\dot{Q}$ ratios in the normal lungs.

During exercise, pulmonary pressure rises so that the distribution of blood flow becomes more uniform and the contribution of the upper zones of the lung to gas exchange is enhanced.

The ventilation/perfusion distribution can be measured by a multiple inert gas method. Areas of high ventilation/low perfusion (high $\dot{V}/\dot{Q}$ ratio) can be regarded as dead space, while areas of low ventilation/high perfusion (low $\dot{V}/\dot{Q}$ ratio) represent venous admixture (physiological shunt).

Pulmonary vascular tone

Both sympathetic and parasympathetic pathways are present in the pulmonary circulation. Noradrenaline causes α_1 adrenoceptor-mediated vasoconstriction, while acetylcholine causes NO-mediated vasodilatation.

Hypoxia causes pulmonary vasoconstriction. Both alveolar and mixed venous oxygen partial pressure play a role in the development of hypoxic vasoconstriction. Because of the influence of alveolar oxygen partial pressure, hypoxic

vasoconstriction may be limited to areas of poor ventilation, thus diverting blood away from poorly ventilated lung, thereby minimising venous admixture. The exact mechanisms of pulmonary hypoxic vasoconstriction have not been elucidated. A number of substances, including hydrogen peroxide (H_2O_2) and arachidonic acid metabolites (eicosanoids), appear to play a role. In addition, K^+ channels may be inhibited by hypoxia. This may lead to depolarisation and increased calcium influx through voltage-activated Ca^{2+} channels.

Numerous pulmonary endothelial mediators have been identified. Endothelium-derived relaxing factor (EDRF, i.e. nitric oxide, NO) is a highly diffusible gas with water and lipid solubilities similar to those of oxygen. NO is inactivated by binding to haemoglobin. Therefore NO is only a vasodilator in the immediate vicinity of its production site. This property of inactivation by haemoglobin makes NO a unique pulmonary vasodilator when administered as a component of inspired gases: pulmonary vasodilatation occurs only in areas that are ventilated. Its administration therefore decreases pulmonary vascular resistance and improves gas exchange. By contrast, pulmonary vasodilators administered systemically may increase blood flow in poorly ventilated lung, thereby increasing venous admixture.

Coronary circulation

Unlike any other organ or tissue, the heart has to provide its own blood supply through the coronary circulation. The coronary vessels are subjected to marked, cyclic variations of extravascular compressive forces, related to the development of tension in the walls of the ventricles. As the myocardium is almost entirely dependent on aerobic metabolism, oxygen demand must be met on a beat-to-beat basis: oxygen extraction approaches 70% at rest. As a result, increases in myocardial oxygen consumption have to be matched by commensurate increases in coronary blood flow. The relationship between coronary blood flow and myocardial oxygen consumption is linear and both coronary sinus oxygen saturation (30%) and oxygen partial pressure (2.6–3.0 kPa) remain remarkably constant in the face of varying oxygen demand.

The right and left coronary arteries arise from the coronary ostia in the sinuses of Valsalva; they run along the atrioventricular grooves. The left coronary artery divides into the left anterior descending and the circumflex arteries. The left anterior descending coronary artery supplies the anterior walls of both ventricles and most of the septum. The circumflex coronary artery supplies the left atrium, part of the posterior wall of the left ventricle, and the sinus node in about 45% of hearts. The right coronary artery supplies the remainder of the right ventricle, the atrioventricular node in about 90% of hearts, and the sino-atrial node in about 55% of hearts. The right coronary artery is often dominant, giving blood supply to the posterior interventricular artery, thus supplying a large proportion of the ventricular myocardium.

From the large epicardial arteries, branches penetrate the myocardium at right-angles and divide into an extensive network of small arteries, which in turn give rise to a very dense capillary network. Branches supplying the subepicardial layers and those supplying the subendocardium are controlled by different mechanisms, so that the transmural distribution of blood flow may vary. Inter- and intracoronary collaterals exist at all levels of vessel size, except the capillaries; further collaterals develop with ischaemia.

Venous return is through coronary veins that drain into the coronary sinus and the right atrium. Some of the venous return from the right ventricle drains into the anterior cardiac vein, which in turn drains directly into the right atrium.

Cerebral circulation

The principal arterial flow to the human brain is carried by two internal carotid and two vertebral arteries. The latter unite to form the basilar artery. The circle of Willis is formed by the internal carotid and the basilar arteries and is the origin of the six large vessels supplying the cerebral cortex, namely the anterior, middle, and posterior cerebral arteries. Venous drainage of the brain is through deep veins and dural sinuses that empty into the internal jugular veins.

Cerebral vessels are innervated by postganglionic sympathetic fibres with neurones in the superior cervical ganglia. The nerve endings contain noradrenaline and neuropeptide Y. There is also cholinergic innervation, principally on large arteries. Only water, CO_2, and O_2 enter the brain easily, while the exchange of other substances is slow. The site of this diffusion barrier is the endothelium of the cerebral capillaries, which constitutes the blood–brain barrier. The blood–brain barrier helps to maintain the constancy of the environment of the neurones in the central nervous system.

The average blood flow in young adults is 54 ml/100 g/min; as the average weight of the brain is 1400 g, flow for the whole brain is about 756 ml/min. Measurement of total cerebral blood flow is possible using the uptake of subanaesthetic concentrations of nitrous oxide (N_2O) as described by Kety-Schmidt.

Blood flow is not uniform throughout the brain – it is higher in the grey matter (69 ml/100 g/min) than in the white matter (28 ml/100 g/min); it is also exquisitely dependent upon the activity of the neurones. Magnetic resonance imaging (MRI) with computed tomography (CT) is used to determine regional cerebral blood flow and draw conclusions as to the exact function of specific areas of the brain.

Regulation of cerebral blood flow

The factors affecting total cerebral blood flow are the arterial pressure, the venous pressure (both taken at brain level), the intracranial pressure, the blood viscosity, and the degree of active vasomotor tone of the cerebral vasculature. The calibre of the cerebral vessels is controlled by local vasodilator metabolites, autoregulatory mechanisms, endothelium-derived mediators, circulating peptides, and vasomotor nerves. Among local vasodilator metabolites, K^+, H^+, and adenosine play a role. In addition, cerebral vessels are very sensitive to changes in O_2 and CO_2 partial pressures. Hypocarbia causes cerebral vasoconstriction, while hypoxia causes vasodilatation. Hypercarbia causes vasodilatation and hyperoxia causes mild vasoconstriction. The cerebral circulation is autoregulated over the range of 65–140 mmHg of cerebral perfusion pressure: cerebral blood flow remains unchanged in the face of large variations in perfusion pressure (Figure 1.12). The autoregulatory curve is shifted towards higher values by sympathetic stimulation and in patients with hypertensive heart disease. This shift means that larger increases in blood pressure can occur without an increase in flow. Conversely, vasodilators reduce the length of the plateau of autoregulation. Increases in P_{CO_2} cause almost-linear increases in cerebral blood flow. Hypoxia also causes increases in cerebral blood flow when P_{O_2} becomes less than approximately 6 kPa (Figure 1.12).

Renal circulation

The renal circulation is complex. Capillaries of the glomeruli are supplied by an afferent and drained by an efferent arteriole. Blood and glomerular filtrate are separated by the capillary endothelium, the basal lamina, and the specialised epithelium that lies on top of the glomerular capillaries. Mesanginal cells lying between basal lamina and endothelium are contractile cells that play a role in the regulation of glomerular filtration. The endothelial cells of the glomerular capillaries are fenestrated with pores 70–90 nm in diameter. The cells have pseudopodia forming filtration slits.

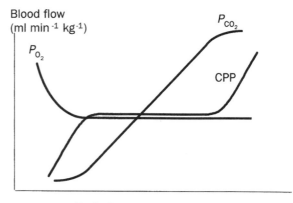

Blood flow (ml min^{-1} kg^{-1})

Perfusion pressure, P_{CO_2}, or P_{O_2}

Figure 1.12 *Schematic representation of the effect of changes in P_{CO_2} and P_{O_2} on cerebral blood flow, superimposed on an autoregulation curve (CPP). The inflection points for autoregulation are 50 and 150 mmHg, for $P_{O_2} \approx 6.5$ kPa, while there is a linear relationship between cerebral blood flow and P_{CO_2}; its intercept with the autoregulation curve occurs at a P_{CO_2} of 5.3 kPa.*

The efferent arterioles break up into capillaries that supply the tubules (peritubular capillaries); these drain into interlobular and renal veins. The afferent arterioles of juxtamedullary glomeruli also form hairpin loops (vasa recta), which are in the immediate vicinity of the loops of Henle. The total surface of the renal capillaries (about 12 m^2) is approximately equal to the total surface area of the tubules.

Renal nerves travel along the renal blood vessels and contain many postganglionic sympathetic fibres. The origin of the sympathetic innervation comes from the lower thoracic and upper lumbar segments of the spinal cord. Sympathetic fibres innervate afferent and efferent arterioles, proximal and distal tubules, and the juxtaglomerular cells.

In a resting adult, the kidneys receive approximately 25% of the cardiac output. Blood flow is much greater in the cortex than in the medulla, as the cortex accounts for approximately 93% of total renal blood flow. Pressure in the glomerular capillaries is approximately 45 mmHg when the mean systemic arterial pressure is 100 mmHg and is only 8 mmHg in the peritubular capillaries. This large difference is due to the resistance of the efferent arteriole.

Renal blood flow is autoregulated such that renal vascular resistance varies with the perfusion pressure to maintain an essentially constant flow rate over a large range of perfusion pressures. Autoregulation is present in denervated kidneys, and is produced in part by direct contractile response of the vascular smooth muscle of the afferent arterioles. At low perfusion pressure, angiotensin II constricts the efferent arterioles, thereby maintaining glomerular filtration.

Catecholamines cause vasoconstriction mainly of interlobular and afferent arterioles; angiotension II constricts the efferent arterioles while prostaglandins increase blood flow in the renal cortex and decrease it in the renal medulla. Acetylcholine produces renal vasodilatation. Sympathetic activation decreases renal blood flow. This effect is mediated by α_1 adrenoceptors and to a lesser extent by postsynaptic α_2 adrenoceptors. Renal vasoconstriction occurs in response to hypotension; this effect is mediated by the baroreceptors. Another effect of sympathetic activation is the stimulation of renin release, mediated by β_1 adrenoceptors, as the juxtaglomerular cells are richly innervated.

Splanchnic circulation

The blood from the intestines, pancreas, and spleen drains via the portal vein into the liver and from the liver via the hepatic veins into the inferior vena cava. The viscera and the liver receive 30% of the cardiac output through the coeliac, superior mesenteric, and inferior mesenteric arteries. The liver receives blood from the hepatic artery (one-third) and the portal vein (two-thirds). Blood flow to the intestines goes predominantly to the mucosa, where it responds to changes in metabolic activity. Blood flow to the small intestine doubles after a meal.

The hepatic circulation is characterised by the presence of large fenestrations in the walls of the hepatic sinusoids, offering high permeability. Sinusoids receive blood from branches of the hepatic artery and the portal vein. They drain into the central lobular veins, the hepatic veins, and finally the inferior vena cava.

The portal venous system is normally a low-pressure system (10 mmHg), yet it converges in the sinusoids with branches of the hepatic artery with a pressure of 90 mmHg. This is possible because there is a marked pressure drop along the hepatic arterioles. This pressure drop is adjusted by the rate of release of adenosine, such that a reduction in portal flow increases flow through the hepatic arteries.

The intrahepatic segments of the portal vein have smooth muscle in their walls. They are innervated by noradrenergeic vasoconstrictor fibres (3rd to 11th thoracic roots, and splanchnic nerves). The vasoconstrictor innervation of the hepatic artery comes from the hepatic sympathetic plexus. In severe shock, liver blood flow is considerably decreased.

The reservoir function of the splanchnic circulation is extensive. Contraction of the capacitance vessels can deliver a litre of blood into the arterial circulation in less than one minute.

Fetal and placental circulations

Blood flow to the uterus is a function of its metabolic requirements and varies with the menstrual cycle. Blood flow increases during pregnancy as the artery increases in size. While arterial blood flow increases 20-fold during pregnancy, metabolic demands of the growing fetus increase much more, and consequently, oxygen extraction increases considerably in the later phase of pregnancy.

The placenta's circulation consists of a maternal portion, a large blood sinus, and a fetal portion containing in its villi small branches of the fetal umbilical arteries and veins. In the placenta, exchange of O_2 and CO_2 is similar to that in the lung, except that O_2 diffusion is less efficient because of the thickness of the cellular layers covering the villi. The placenta, in addition to O_2 uptake and CO_2 release, serves as entry port for all nutrients, and exit port for all fetal waste products.

In the fetus, 55% of the cardiac output goes through the placenta (Figure 1.13). The blood returning from the placenta in the umbilical vein is 80% saturated. Some of this blood is diverted directly into the inferior vena cava through the

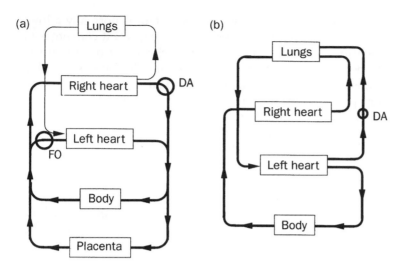

Figure 1.13 *Diagrammatic representation of the fetal circulation (a) and the circulation shortly after birth (b). FO, foramen ovale; DA, ductus arteriosus. Once the ductus arteriosus is closed, the two circulations become fully coupled (not represented).*

ductus venosus. The remainder mixes with the portal blood of the fetus. Portal and systemic venous blood is only 25% saturated. Admixture with blood from the umbilical vein brings saturation to 67%. Most of the venous return is diverted through the open foramen ovale into the left atrium. The blood returning through the superior vena cava enters the right ventricle and, because of the high resistance of the pulmonary vasculature, most of it passes into the aorta through the open ductus arteriosus. From the aorta, blood circulates to the placenta and into body tissues.

At birth, the placental circulation is interrupted and peripheral vascular resistance increases. Pressure in the aorta exceeds pressure in the pulmonary artery. As the lungs expand at delivery, the pulmonary vascular resistance decreases to one-fifth of its value in utero. The sudden increase in pulmonary blood flow in response to the much lower pulmonary vascular resistance causes an increase in left atrial pressure, which closes the foramen ovale. At the same time, the ductus arteriosus constricts so that an adult-type circulation is established. Bradykinin constricts the umbilical vessels and the ductus arteriosus, and causes pulmonary vasodilatation. It may play a role in the transition from fetal to adult circulation.

FURTHER READING

Andersen MC. Nucleus tractus solitarius – gateway to neural circulatory control. *Annu Rev Physiol* 1994; **56**: 96–113.

Atlee JL. Perioperative cardiac dysrhythmias: diagnostic and management. *Anesthesiology* 1997; **86**: 1397–424.

Bahkle YS. Pharmacokinetic and metabolic properties of the lung. *Br J Anaesthesia* 1990; **65**: 79–93.

Balser JR, Atlee JL. Cardiac electrophysiology. In: *Foundations of Anaesthesia. Basic and Clinical Sciences.* (Hemmings H Jr, Hopkins PM, eds). London: Mosby, 2000: 371–80.

Berne RM, Levy MN. *Cardiovascular Physiology* 7th edn. St Louis, MO: Mosby, 1997.

Brady AJ. Mechanical properties of isolated cardiac myocytes. *Physiol Rev* 1991; **71**: 413–42.

Calver A, Collier J, Vallance P. Nitric oxide and cardiovascular control. *Exp Physiol* 1993; **78**: 303–26.

Cannell MB, Cheng H, Lederer WJ. The control of calcium release in heart muscle. *Science* 1995; **268**; 1045–9.

Faraci FM, Heistad DD. Regulation of the cerebral circulation: role of endothelium and potassium channels. *Physiol Rev* 1998; **78**: 53–74.

Feigl EO. Coronary physiology. *Physiol Rev* 1983; **63**: 1–205.

Fuchs F. Mechanical modulation of the Ca²⁺ regulatory protein complex in cardiac muscle. *News Physiol Sci* 1995; **10**: 6–12.

Grossman JD, Morgan JP. Cardiovascular effects of endothelin. *News Physiol Sci* 1997; **12**: 113–17.

Hainsworth R. Reflexes from the heart. *Physiol Rev* 1991; **71**: 617–58.

Heerdt PM. Regulation and assessment of cardiac function. In: *Foundations of Anaesthesia. Basic and Clinical Sciences.* (Hemmings H Jr, Hopkins PM, eds). London: Mosby, 2000: 381–408.

Jackson WF. Potassium channels and regulation of the microcirculation. *Microcirculation* 1998; **5**: 85–90.

Levick JR. *An Introduction to Cardiovascular Physiology* 3rd edn. London: Arnold, 2000.

Malpas SC, Leonard BL. Neural regulation of renal blood flow: a re-examination. *Clin Exp Pharmacol Physiol* 2000; **27**: 956–64.

Mary DASG. Reflex effects on the coronary circulation. *Exp Physiol* 1992; **77**: 243–70.

Nyhan D, Blanck TJJ. Cardiac physiology. In: *Foundations of Anaesthesia. Basic and Clinical Sciences.* (Hemmings H Jr, Hopkins PM, eds). London: Mosby, 2000: 361–70.

Priebe H-J, Skarvan K (eds). *Cardiovascular Physiology.* London: BMJ Publishing, 1995.

Schadt JC, Ludbrook J. Hemodynamic and neurohumoral reponses to acute hypovolaemia in conscious mammals. *Am J Physiol* 1991; **260**: H305–18.

Spyer KM. Central nervous contribution to cardiovascular control. *J Physiol (Lond)* 1994; **474**: 1–19.

2

Respiratory physiology

Paul CM van den Berg

INTRODUCTION

The primary function of the respiratory system is to effectively manage oxygen uptake and carbon dioxide output. The load imposed on the lung depends on the metabolic activity of the body, and can change over a wide range, primarily influenced by body temperature and muscle activity. The lung has a huge reserve capacity and, despite more than 50-fold changes in oxygen consumption and carbon dioxide production, the arterial and mixed venous blood gases are maintained remarkably constant. The normal range of blood gas tensions is $P_{aCO_2} = 4.8 - 5.9$ kPa and $P_{aO_2} = 11.3 - 13.3$ kPa. The first signs of pulmonary impairment usually manifest during exercise, when the demands on functional capacity are high. Respiratory failure is defined by $P_{aCO_2} > 6.7$ kPa and $P_{aO_2} < 8.0$ kPa (breathing room air) measured at sea level and without metabolic alkalosis.

Oxygen transfer from air to cell depends on the oxygen uptake in the lung and the transport capacity of the blood. Under physiological conditions, oxygen transport is governed primarily by cardiac output. Changing demands for oxygen by the cells parallel changes in left ventricular output. The primary means by which carbon dioxide tension is maintained is by adjustments in minute ventilation.

FUNCTIONAL PULMONARY ANATOMY

The lungs in an adult weigh 900–1000 g. The right lung, with three lobes, is somewhat larger than the left lung, which has two lobes. After a passive expiration, the adult lung contains about 2.5 l of air. With maximum inspiration, the volume increases to approximately 6 l TLC (total lung capacity). The lungs contain stretch receptors that are stimulated with inflation and activate the Hering–Breurer reflex. This reflex causes bronchodilatation, an increase in heart rate, and a decrease in peripheral vascular resistance. Receptors in the epithelium of the trachea cause bronchoconstriction, coughing, and mucus secretion when provoked by mechanical stimulation or by inhaled irritants. During inspiration, air passes first through the nose and/or mouth. In the nose, a complex structure of irregular passages, the turbinates, help trap inhaled particles and warm and humidify the inspired air. Air then passes via the larynx and vocal cords into the trachea, from where it eventually reaches the terminal bronchioles and alveoli, where gas exchange occurs. Alveolar air is fully saturated with water vapour. At 37°C, water vapour pressure is 6.27 kPa. The remaining gases have partial pressures corresponding to their fractional concentrations. The total pressure is atmospheric pressure minus water vapour pressure (101.33 – 6.27 = 95 kPa). Air contains 21% oxygen, and the inspired oxygen tension is therefore $95 \times 21\% = 19.9$ kPa. The other relevant gases in the alveolar space are nitrogen and carbon dioxide. Nitrogen is an inert gas and therefore its inspiratory and alveolar concentrations are identical.

In the alveolus, carbon dioxide is added to the gas mixture and dilutes the oxygen. This means that the oxygen concentration in the alveolus is different from the inspired oxygen concentration. The alveolar oxygen concentration is practically identical to the arterial oxygen concentration, although the difference can become marked by lung or cardiac disease. Under steady-state conditions, the oxygen consumption equals the quantity of oxygen entering the lung by ventilation minus the amount removed in the blood:

$$\dot{V}_{O_2} = \dot{V}_A (F_{IO_2} - F_{AO_2})$$

$$F_{AO_2} = F_{IO_2} - \frac{\dot{V}_A}{\dot{V}_{O_2}}$$

Tracheobronchial tree

The airways beneath the larynx form a tree structure that progressively birfurcates down to the alveolar sacs (Figure 2.1). The largest airway, the trachea, is designated as generation 0. With each bifurcation, the number of airways doubles; 2 main bronchi, 4 lobar bronchi, 16 segmental bronchi, etc. Airways up to generation 5 contain cartilaginous rings; those between generations 6 and 14 are membranous bronchioli. Beyond generation 15, airways not only conduct air but also participate in gas exchange. Although the diameters of each generation decrease, the total cross-sectional area progressively increases (Table 2.1). There are about 300 million alveoli in the human lung, arising from airway generations 17–23. They have a total surface area of approximately 80 m². Their very thin walls (0.1–0.2 μm) allow easy gas exchange between the alveolar air and the pulmonary capillaries.

The airways contain different types of cells. The tracheal mucosa contains ciliated epithelium and numerous mucus-secreting goblet cells. Cilia beat in a coordinated manner to move mucus and inhaled particles towards the pharynx. They are responsible for the mechanical cleaning of the upper airways. The walls of the alveoli contain type I cells, which cover 95% of the alveolar surface, and type II cells which produce surfactant. Surfactant is a mixture of dipalmitoyl phosphatidylcholine (DPPC), other lipids, and a protein that helps stabilise DPPC at the air–liquid interface. According to Laplace's law,

$$P = 2T/r$$

where P is the pressure within the alveolus, T is the surface tension, and r is the radius of curvature, smaller alveoli should collapse into larger ones (Figure 2.2). Surfactant, which lines the alveoli, considerably lowers the surface tension and prevents collapse. Lack or deficiency of surfactant contributes to the atelactasis in hyaline membrane disease in premature infants and in adult (acute) respiratory distress syndrome (ARDS).

LUNG VOLUMES

The lung volume is divided into several overlapping components, which vary between individuals and depend on age, sex, height, and body position. By convention, a volume that cannot be subdivided into smaller components is referred to as a 'volume', and a volume that is a combination of other volumes is called a 'capacity'. The tidal volume V_T is the volume of air that moves in and out of the lungs with each breath. The average tidal volume at rest is about 500 ml in an adult. With normal breathing, the reserve capacities above and below the tidal volume are approximately equal and are called the inspiratory reserve volume IRV and the functional residual capacity FRC (Figure 2.3). IRV is the additional air inspired by a maximum inspiratory effort. The expiratory reserve volume ERV is the additional air expelled by active expiration. The vital capacity VC is the sum ERV + V_T + IRV. FRC is the volume of air in the lungs at the end of a normal expiration with the subject standing, and is about 2.5 l. In the supine position, FRC is reduced to about 1 l, due to movement of the diaphragm caused by upward movement of the abdominal contents. The TLC is the volume of gas in the lung after a maximum inspiration. In the average adult man, TLC

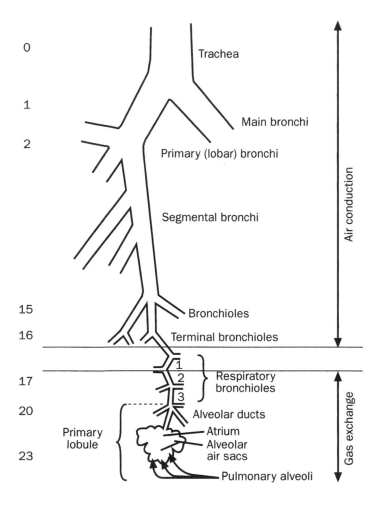

Figure 2.1 Anatomy of the air passages. The numbers on the left are the airway generations.

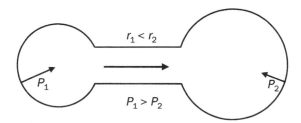

Figure 2.2 Schematic illustration of Laplace's law. Two bubbles of different diameters are connected by a tube. Because of forces due to surface tension, the pressure in the smaller bubble is greater than that in the larger one, with the result that the smaller collapses into the larger. In the lungs, this is prevented by surfactant, which reduces surface tension forces.

is about 6 l. For an adult woman of the same size, the TLC is 5% less: 5.7 l. FRC is the most important capacity in the lung. Most pathological lung conditions are associated with a reduction in FRC. The inspiratory capacity is subdivided into the inspiratory reserve volume IRV and the tidal volume V_T. FRC is subdivided into the expiratory reserve volume ERV and the residual volume RV.

LUNG MECHANICS

Ventilation results from contraction of the respiratory muscles and the forces of elastic recoil of

Table 2.1 Dimensions of the human airways up to the 17th generation

Generation	Diameter (cm)	Total cross-sectional area (cm²)	Total volume (ml)
0	1.8	2.5	30
1	1.2	2.3	42
2	0.76	2.13	46
3	0.56	2.0	47
4	0.45	2.5	51
5	0.35	3.1	54
6	0.28	4.0	57
7	0.23	5.1	61
8	0.19	7.0	66
9	0.15	9.6	80
10	0.13	13.4	77
11	0.11	19.6	85
12	0.09	28.8	94
13	0.08	44.5	106
14	0.074	69.4	122
15	0.066	116.0	145
16	0.06	180.0	175
17	0.054	300.0	218

the lungs and thorax. During inspiration, work is done by the intercostal muscles and the diaphragm to overcome the resistance of the airways and the elastic recoil of lung tissue. During quiet breathing, expiration is normally passive. When the respiratory muscles do not produce external work, the passive forces of the lung, which tend to decrease lung volume, are opposed by the passive mechanical properties of the thoracic wall, which tends to increase intrathoracic volume. The result of these opposing forces is a negative pressure in the pleural cavity when the lung volume is at FRC. The mechanical characteristics of the chest wall affect the resting lung volume and the forces needed to change it. These characteristics are significantly altered by changes in body position. FRC is largest in the erect and least in the prone position, and intermediate in the supine position.

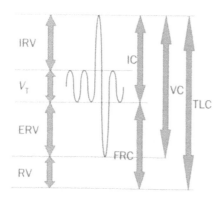

Figure 2.3 *The volumes of the lung: IRV, inspiratory reserve volume; V$_T$, tidal volume; ERV, expiratory reserve volume; RV, reserve volume; IC, inspiratory capacity; FRC, functional residual capacity; VC, vital capacity; TLC, total lung capacity.*

Compliance

The elastic properties of the lung are measured in terms of compliance C, which is the extent to which the lung expands for each unit increase in transpulmonary pressure (the difference between alveolar and intrapleural pressure). Compliance is a measure of the ease of distension of the lungs. It is measured as the slope of the lung volume versus transpulmonary pressure curve (Figure 2.4), with units ml/cmH_2O:

$$C = \frac{\Delta V}{\Delta P}$$

The higher the compliance, the less distension pressure is needed to achieve a given lung volume. The total compliance C_T in the average adult is about 200 ml/cmH₂O. This has two components: lung compliance C_L and chest wall compliance C_{CW}, which have approximately equal values of 200 ml/cmH₂O, and are related to C_T by the following expression (analogous to electrical capacitances):

$$\frac{1}{C_T} = \frac{1}{C_L} + \frac{1}{C_{CW}}$$

Compliance is volume-dependent: a reduction in lung volume, from whatever cause, reduces the compliance of the lung, and vice versa. Parenchymal changes in the lung caused by fibrosis or congestion decrease compliance. Emphysema results in an increase in compliance.

Compliance can be subdivided into static and dynamic compliance. Static compliance is measured after all lung units are filled and the volume at any level in the lung is constant. Dynamic compliance is a measure of the volume and pressure changes that occur during normal breathing. It is calculated from the volume and pressure in the lung measured at zero flow when airflow is blocked for a short moment during a normal respiration. The relationship between static and dynamic compliance depends on the distribution of the time constants of the respiratory units. The difference increases when, due to long time constants,

some units are not completely filled. The difference therefore becomes more marked with increasing respiratory frequency.

Closing capacity

At the end of a passive expiration, the opposing forces of lung recoil and chest wall expansion are in equilibrium, and the intrapleural pressure is least negative. During expiration below FRC, the small airways can collapse and close. The closed airways do not take part in gas exchange, but are still perfused with pulmonary capillary blood, so that oxygenation in these regions is impaired. The volume at which this occurs is the closing capacity. Closing capacity increases with age. In young adults, it is below FRC, and thus does not normally occur during normal tidal breathing. By 65 years, closure of basal airways occurs during normal tidal breathing in the erect position. This is one of the reasons why arterial P_{O_2} decreases with age. The closing capacity is less in the supine than in the erect position, and by the age of 45 years encroaches on FRC in the supine position.

Airway resistance

Apart from elastic forces, ventilation has to overcome airway resistance, which accounts for approximately 30% of the work of breathing at rest. More than 50% of airway resistance arises in the upper airways and less than 10% is due to the peripheral airways. The pressure drop between mouth and alveoli is 0.5–2.0 kPa at a flow rate of 1 l/min. As the diameter of the airways increases with increasing lung volume, the resistance declines exponentially. The airway diameter changes between inspiration and expiration. During inspiration, the negative intrapleural pressure increases the airway diameter. During expiration, positive intrapleural pressure decreases the diameter. Narrowing of the airway during expiration is an important mechanism for increasing flow in the airways to very high levels during coughing. The cough reflex is triggered by mechanical stimuli arising in the larynx, trachea, carina, and main bronchi. When the closed glottis opens, a forced expiration

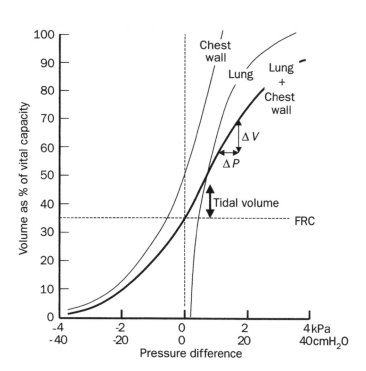

Figure 2.4 *Compliance curves for the lung and the chest wall and the combined curve.*

through narrowed airways creates a high flow velocity and sweeps irritant material up towards the pharynx.

Time constants

The combined mechanical properties of lung compliance and airways resistance are best described by the time constant of the alveolus. The time constant τ of an alveolus is defined as the time it takes to fill when a constant pressure is applied. The filling process is exponential, so that after τ, 63% of the final volume is reached; after 2τ, 87%, and after 4τ, 98% is attained. The time constant equals the product of resistance and compliance:

$$\tau = RC$$

Under physiological conditions, there is a narrow range of time constants, but the range increases with many lung diseases. Under pathological conditions, τ may increase to a level that prevents unrestricted volume change. Ventilation in these units decreases and becomes highly dependent on respiratory rate. The higher the respiratory rate, the lower the measured dynamic compliance.

WORK OF BREATHING

The work of breathing is determined by the product of transpulmonary pressure (driving pressure) and volume change (tidal volume). This can be expressed mathematically as:

$$\int P \, dV$$

which is the hatched area under the pressure–volume loop in Figure 2.5. The work of breathing varies between 2.5 and 4 J/min (~ 0.5 J/l). Ventilation requires work to overcome two components, elastic work (stretching the lungs and chest wall) and frictional work to overcome airway resistance. Elastic work requires 75% of total respiratory work and resistive work 25%. During quiet breathing, almost all work is done during inspiration, as expiration is passive, and the total energy needed for ventilation accounts for only 1–3% of oxygen consumption. This can increase up to 50-fold during strenuous exercise.

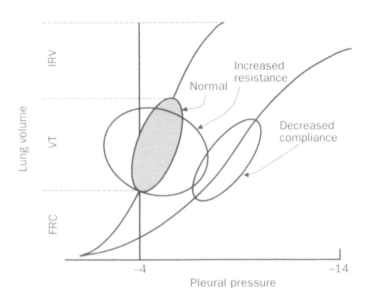

Figure 2.5 *Pressure–volume curves for a normal lung and one with decreased compliance. Superimposed on the curves are pressure–volume loops for the normal situation, decreased compliance, and increased airway resistance. The hatched loop represents the work of breathing.*

A decrease in compliance or an increase in airway resistance can also dramatically increase the work of breathing. Under these conditions, the respiratory pattern is adjusted in an attempt to obtain the maximum ventilation for the least energy expenditure. When the compliance of the lung is low, the respiratory rate increases so that the small tidal volume falls within the steep part of the compliance curve. In contrast, when the airway resistance is increased, it is beneficial to decrease the respiratory rate in an attempt to decrease flow and respiratory work.

VENTILATION AND GAS EXCHANGE

The anatomy of the lungs dictates that a portion of each breath does not take part in gas exchange. This anatomical dead space comprises the larger airways that have to be passed before air reaches the respiratory units where gas exchange takes place. The anatomical dead space is 2–3 ml/kg. It can be measured from a graph of carbon dioxide concentration at the lips against exhaled volume (Figure 2.6). A mismatch between alveolar ventilation and perfusion also contributes to a dead-space effect: the alveolar dead space. This is very small in a healthy individual. The sum of anatomical and alveolar dead space is called the physiological

dead space V_D. Usually this is expressed as a ratio V_D/V_T, and is normally about 30%, but is increased in lung disease. An increase in V_D/V_T, equivalent to rebreathing, results in an increase in alveolar carbon dioxide. The respiratory system responds with an increase in minute ventilation until the elevated carbon dioxide tension is normalized. However, this requires an increase in the work of breathing. When V_D/V_T increases above 60%, the respiratory work needed to maintain normocapnia cannot be maintained and hypercapnia ensues. V_D/V_T can be calculated using the Bohr equation:

$$\frac{V_D}{V_T} = \frac{P_{aCO_2} - P_{ECO_2}}{P_{aCO_2}}$$

CARBON DIOXIDE EXCHANGE

Carbon dioxide production is a function of the respiratory quotient R and oxygen consumption:

$$R = \frac{\text{rate of } CO_2 \text{ production}}{\text{rate of } O_2 \text{ consumption}}$$

Under resting conditions, carbon dioxide production is 200 ml/min and oxygen consumption 250 ml/min, giving a value for R of 0.8, but this

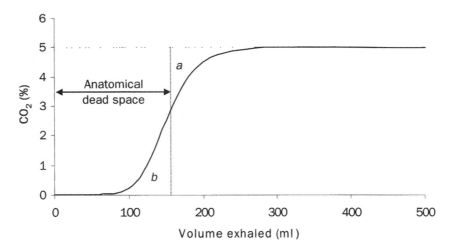

Figure 2.6 *Fowler's graphical method for measuring anatomical dead space from a plot of expired CO_2 concentration versus expired volume. The anatomical dead space is the volume for which the areas* a *and* b *are equal.*

is dependent on the type of metabolic substrate. R for fat is 0.7 and R is 1 for carbohydrates. During steady state, the production of carbon dioxide equals the amount excreted by the lungs:

$$\dot{V}_{CO_2} = \dot{V}_A F_{ACO_2} = \dot{V}_E F_{ECO_2}$$

Rearranging,

$$F_{ACO_2} = \frac{\dot{V}_{CO_2}}{\dot{V}_A}$$

and

$$P_{ACO_2} = F_{ACO_2} = (P_B - P_{H_2O})$$

Substituting gives the alveolar ventilation equation:

$$P_{ACO_2} = \frac{\dot{V}_{CO_2}}{\dot{V}_A}(P_B - P_{H_2O})$$

This equation relates alveolar carbon dioxide tension and alveolar ventilation (Figure 2.7). The alveolar ventilation is under direct control of the respiratory centre in the brainstem, which controls the carbon dioxide concentration in the blood within narrow limits. The largest source

of carbon dioxide production is muscle activity. Each degree Celsius change in body temperature changes carbon dioxide production by 14%.

Carbon dioxide transport

The solubility of carbon dioxide in the blood is about 24 times greater than the solubility of oxygen (0.072 ml/dl/mmHg versus 0.003 ml/dl/mmHg), so that much more is transported in the dissolved form. Carbon dioxide is stored in the blood in three forms: in physical solution, protein-bound as carbamino, and as bicarbonate. Carbon dioxide binds with blood proteins, in particular haemoglobin, to form carbamino compounds:

$$R - NH_2 + CO_2 \leftrightarrow R - NH - COO^- + H^+$$

Despite its high solubility, dissolved carbon dioxide represents only 6% of the total arterial carbon dioxide content under normal conditions. Carbamino compounds account for a further 4% and the remainder is stored as bicarbonate. The formation of bicarbonate depends on the enzyme carbonic anhydrase (CA), which catalyses the rapid conversion of carbon dioxide to bicarbonate:

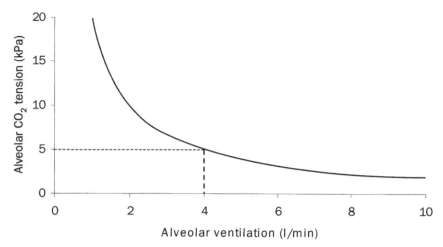

Figure 2.7 *The hyperbolic relationship between alveolar ventilation and alveolar CO$_2$ tension.*

$$CO_2 + H_2O \overset{CA}{\rightarrow} H_2CO_3 \rightarrow H^+ + HCO_3^-$$

When carbon dioxide binds to haemoglobin in the tissues, it reduces its affinity for oxygen, making the latter more readily available to the cells. This is known as the *Bohr effect*. The opposite occurs in the lungs, where the increasing oxygen saturation shifts the carbon dioxide dissociation curve to the right, releasing carbon dioxide (the *Haldane effect*). The carbon dioxide dissociation curve is much more linear than that of oxygen, and in the range 4.5–6.5 kPa is almost a straight line. The Haldane effect makes the physiological dissociation curve steeper than a curve measured in vitro (Figure 2.8).

EXCHANGE MECHANISMS FOR OXYGEN

The oxygen stores in the body are small compared with oxygen consumption. This is especially accentuated when oxygen consumption increases due to muscle activity. When breathing air ($F_{iO_2} = 0.21$) the oxygen stored in the lung at FRC is 400 ml. One litre of oxygen is dissolved in blood and about 200 ml is dissolved in the body tissues. The amount of oxygen delivered to the body is the product of cardiac output and the arterial oxygen content and is around 1000 ml/min in an adult. The normal oxygen consumption is about 250 ml/min. Consequently, three-quarters of the oxygen delivered to the tissues is returned to the lung.

The oxygen tension in an alveolus depends on the amount of oxygen delivered by ventilation and the quantity removed by the blood. The former is a function of the inspired oxygen concentration and alveolar ventilation. The quantity removed depends on pulmonary blood flow and the oxygen-carrying capacity of the blood. Oxygen is carried in the blood mainly in association with haemoglobin, with only a small amount dissolved in the plasma (0.3 ml/dl). In contrast, each 100 ml blood has an oxygen-carrying capacity of 1.36 ml/g haemoglobin. With a haemoglobin concentration of 15 g/dl and a P_{aO_2} of 13 kPa, each 100 ml blood carries approximately 20 ml oxygen combined with haemoglobin and 0.3 ml of dissolved oxygen:

$$C_{aO_2} = 0.0225P_{O_2} + 1.36S_{aO_2}Hb$$

where 0.0225 ml/dl/kPa is the solubility coefficient of oxygen. The resting oxygen consumption is approximately 250 ml/min. The relationship between oxygen consumption, oxygen content and cardiac output is given by the Fick equation:

$$\dot{V}_{O_2} = CO(C_{aO_2} - C_{vO_2})$$

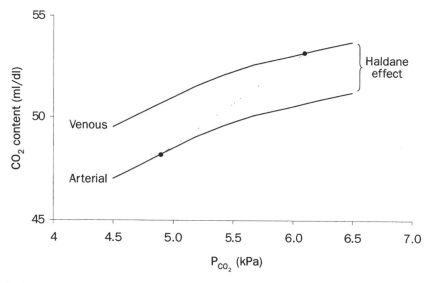

Figure 2.8 *CO_2–haemoglobin dissociation curve, illustrating the Haldane effect.*

The term in parentheses is the arteriovenous difference, which with normal oxygen consumption is about 5 ml/dl. It is a good indicator of the adequacy of oxygen delivery to the tissues. The Fick equation can be used to calculate cardiac output, by measuring oxygen consumption and mixed venous oxygen content. For this application C_{aO_2} is the oxygen content in the pulmonary venous blood, which is difficult to obtain, but in the absence of significant shunting can be taken as 20 ml/dl with little loss of accuracy.

The oxygen–haemoglobin dissociation curve

The reason that the arteriovenous difference plays a crucial role in the delivery of oxygen to the tissues depends to a large extent on the shape of the oxygen dissociation curve. The affinity of haemoglobin for oxygen is nonlinear, the characteristic sigmoid shape of the oxygen dissociation curve (Figure 2.9) reflecting the complex interaction between oxygen and the four protein subunits of the iron–porphyrin haem moiety. The ferrous iron of haem forms a loose reversible complex with oxygen, each molecule of haemoglobin binding with up to four molecules of oxygen. However, the affinity for oxygen increases as it combines with more molecules of haem.

The position of the oxygen dissociation curve is defined by P_{50}, the P_{O_2} at which haemoglobin is 50% saturated. The normal P_{50} is 3.5 kPa (26 mmHg). The main factors governing the position of the haemoglobin dissociation curve are pH, P_{CO_2}, temperature, and 2,3-diphosphoglycerate (DPG) concentration. DPG is an intermediate product of red cell glycolysis. It binds to the β chains of haemoglobin, reducing its affinity for oxygen. An increase in DPG concentration increases the unloading of oxygen from haemoglobin, facilitating the supply of oxygen to the tissues. DPG production is increased by exposure to high altitudes and by anaemia. Factors that increase P_{50} (acidosis or increased P_{CO_2}; the Bohr effect) shift the dissociation curve to the right, reduce the affinity of haemoglobin for oxygen, and encourage oxygen release. This occurs in the tissues. The opposite occurs in the lungs when the decrease in P_{50} causes a shift to the left, allowing more oxygen to bind to haemoglobin. Here the attachment of oxygen to haem reduces the capacity of haemoglobin to bind CO_2 (the Haldane effect), facilitating its elimination by the lungs.

The steep part of the dissociation curve falls between P_{O_2} values of 1 and 8 kPa. In this range, a change in oxygen tension causes the greatest change in oxygen saturation. At the normal P_{aO_2}

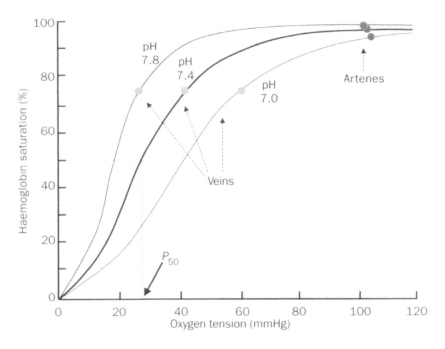

Figure 2.9 *O_2–haemoglobin dissociation curve for different pH values.*

haemoglobin is 98% saturated and increasing P_{aO_2} above about 14 kPa produces little change in saturation, since beyond this tension the dissociation curve is flat. The saturation begins to fall steeply as P_{aO_2} decreases below about 8 kPa. This facilitates release of oxygen to the tissues. Mixed venous blood has a P_{O_2} of 5.3 kPa and a saturation of 75%.

VENTILATION–PERFUSION INEQUALITY

At rest, the alveolar ventilation $\dot{V}_A$ in a healthy adult is about 4–4.5 l/min and the pulmonary blood flow $\dot{Q}$ is 5 l/min. This gives a global ventilation/perfusion ratio $\dot{V}/\dot{Q}$ of 0.8–0.9. During spontaneous breathing, however, ventilation and perfusion are not evenly distributed over the lung. In the erect position, hydrostatic forces cause an increase in intrapleural pressure from the top to the bottom of the lung, by approximately 0.2–0.4 cmH$_2$O/cm distance. This positions dependent regions on the lower, steeper part of the pressure–volume curve. Since during inspiration transpulmonary pressure (airway pressure minus intrapleural pressure) increases equally over the lung, dependent regions are better ventilated than non-dependent ones (Figure 2.10). Dependent regions also receive a greater blood flow, due to the influence of gravity. The decrease in blood flow from the top to the bottom of the lung is much more than the fall in ventilation. The lung can be divided into three zones (West's lung zones), depending on alveolar, arterial, and pulmonary venous pressures (Figure 2.11). In the upper region (zone 1), $P_A > P_a > P_v$, and alveoli in this zone are over-ventilated in relationship to their perfusion. In the intermediate part of the lung (zone 2), $P_a > P_A > P_v$. Zone 3 is the lower part of the lung, where $P_a > P_v > P_A$ and alveoli are overperfused in relationship to their ventilation. This mismatch between ventilation and perfusion reduces the efficiency of gas exchange. In areas where the ventilation–perfusion ratio is high, alveolar P_{O_2} is high and P_{CO_2} is low (functional dead space). Where the ratio is low (shunt), P_{O_2} is low and P_{CO_2} high (Figure 2.12). Shunt is the passage of deoxygenated blood from the venous

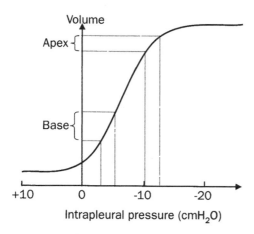

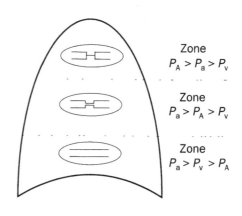

Figure 2.10 *Volume–pressure curve showing the variation in volume changes for the same change in intrapleural pressure between the apex and the base of the lung.*

Figure 2.11 *West's three lung zones for distribution of pulmonary blood flow and alveolar ventilation.*

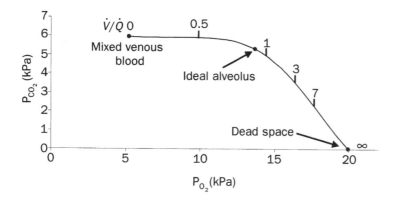

Figure 2.12 *O_2–CO_2 diagram showing the possible values of P_{O_2} and P_{CO_2} in the blood for all possible values of venous admixture.*

circulation to the arterial side of the circulation without picking up oxygen (Figure 2.13). Physiological shunting occurs from two anatomical sources: bronchial circulation that drains into the pulmonary veins, and the Thesbian veins that drain from the walls of the left ventricle directly into the left ventricle. Normally these anatomical sources account for less than 1.5% of cardiac output, but this may increase in lung diseases. The most common causes of intrapulmonary shunt are atelectasis, pulmonary oedema, and consolidation. Extreme shunting occurs in areas of atelactesis that are perfused but not ventilated ($\dot{V}/\dot{Q} = 0$).

Venous admixture, often simply referred to as 'shunt', consists of true anatomical shunts plus shunt due to ventilation–perfusion heterogenicity in the lung. Venous admixture is the calculated admixture of mixed venous blood with pulmonary end-capillary blood that would be required to produce the observed difference between the arterial and pulmonary end-capillary P_{O_2}. The latter is usually taken as equal to ideal alveolar P_{O_2}. The concept of ideal alveolar air was developed to quantify the inefficiency of oxygen gas exchange. If there were no barrier to the diffusion of gases and no ventilation–perfusion inequalities, the arterial and alveolar oxygen

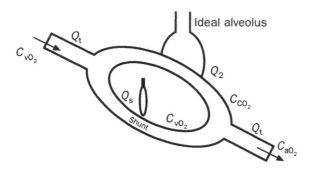

Figure 2.13 *Cartoon illustrating shunting in the lung.*

tensions would be equal, as would the carbon dioxide tensions. The ideal alveolar P_{O_2} represents the P_{O_2} that would exist in a perfectly ventilated and perfused lung exchanging gas at the respiratory exchange ratio. 'Ideal' alveolar gas cannot be sampled, but its P_{O_2} can be calculated from the alveolar air equation:

$$P_{AO_2} = P_{IO_2} - P_{aCO_2} \frac{P_{IO_2} - P_{EO_2}}{P_{EO_2}}$$

The shunt fraction is defined as the ratio between shunted blood and total cardiac output. This is calculated from the Berggren shunt equation. The basis of this equation is that the total oxygen content of blood leaving the left ventricle is the sum of oxygen content in the pulmonary end-capillary blood flow and the oxygen content in the shunted blood:

$$\dot{Q}_t C_{aO_2} = \dot{Q}_s C_{vO_2} + (\dot{Q}_t - \dot{Q}_s) C'_{cO_2}$$

Rearranging this equation gives the shunt equation:

$$\frac{\dot{Q}_s}{\dot{Q}_t} = \frac{C'_{cO_2} - C_{aO_2}}{C'_{cO_2} - C_{vO_2}}$$

The mixed venous oxygen content represents the average oxygen content of blood returned to the lung. It can be measured in blood from the pulmonary artery, or calculated assuming an arteriovenous oxygen content difference of 5 vol%. The arterial oxygen content can be easily measured, or taken as 20 ml per 100 ml blood in a healthy individual breathing air. The capillary oxygen content is calculated from the alveolar air equation assuming equality between capillary and alveolar oxygen tension.

Although alveoli with a high ventilation–perfusion ratio can compensate for those with low ratios, this carries a high price. Hyperventilated alveoli are much less efficient than underventilated alveoli. In hyperventilated alveoli the carbon dioxide concentration is low so that, for a particular alveolar ventilation, less carbon dioxide is output than in hypoventilated alveoli with a high carbon dioxide concentration. Further, the blood flow to hyperventilated units is usually far less than that to hypoventilated units. Together this leads to minimum gain in carbon dioxide output at a high cost in respiratory work. Consequently, the carbon dioxide concentration in the blood rises when respiratory muscles fail and minute ventilation diminishes. A new equilibrium is attained when the carbon dioxide concentration in the alveoli increases to a level where production and output match.

Alveolar-to-arterial oxygen pressure difference $P_{(A-a)O_2}$

In a healthy young adult breathing air, the alveolar–arterial oxygen tension difference $P_{(A-a)O_2}$ is less than 0.7 kPa. but may rise to 5 kPa in the healthy elderly individual. Any lung disease that causes venous admixture will increase $P_{(A-a)O_2}$. While an increase in dead space can be compensated for by an increase in minute ventilation, increased venous admixture inevitably leads to hypoxaemia. This is due to the shape of the haemoglobin saturation curve and because the oxygen saturation is normally close to 100% (Figure 2.9). The relationship between $P_{(A-a)O_2}$ and calculated shunt is altered by changes in F_{iO_2}. Delivering more oxygen to an alveolus with a low ventilation–perfusion ratio will increase the oxygen tension in the arterial blood. Note, however, that it is only possible to compensate for hypoxaemia due to venous admixture by increasing F_{iO_2} when the shunt fraction is less than about 30%, and this may require 100% inspired oxygen.

$P_{(A-a)O_2}$ is affected by several factors apart from venous admixture. It increases by approximately 1 kPa for each 10% increase in F_{iO_2}. To circumvent this problem, the evaluation of lung function based on oxygen tension in arterial blood is best evaluated with the P_{aO_2}/F_{iO_2} ratio. Under physiological conditions, the ratio is greater than 450, but in severe lung disease, it can drop to below 200. The relationship between shunt and $P_{(A-a)O_2}$ is also influenced considerably by cardiac output, oxygen consumption, and, to a lesser extent, by haemoglobin concentration, carbon dioxide tension, temperature, and acid–base status. In the shunt equation above, C_{aO_2} - C_{vO_2} is the arterial/mixed venous oxygen content difference. This is related to cardiac output and oxygen consumption by the Fick equation (see above). Changes in cardiac output produce inverse changes in C_{aO_2} - C_{vO_2}, provided that oxygen consumption remains constant.

Because of the shape of the oxygen dissociation curve, a small increase in F_{iO_2} may result in a significant increase in haemoglobin saturation when the saturation is low. This sensitivity to small increases in F_{iO_2} is the rationale behind oxygen therapy. It may also be used to distinguish between venous admixture and ventilation–perfusion inequality. When breathing 100% oxygen, the decrease in $P_{(A-a)O_2}$ is linearly related to shunt up to 25–30% since the oxygen dissociation curve is virtually flat for $P_{O_2} > 25$ kPa. A general rule of thumb is that every 1% shunt causes a 2 kPa increase in $P_{(A-a)O_2}$, provided that cardiac output, and thus C_{aO_2} - C_{vO_2}, is normal.

CONTROL OF BREATHING

The respiratory centre in the medulla controls the rate and volume of ventilation, modulated by feedback loops from central and peripheral chemoreceptors that sense blood P_{CO_2}, P_{O_2}, and hydrogen ion concentration. About 80% of the respiratory response to carbon dioxide comes from the central chemoreceptors, and the remainder from the peripheral receptors. The neurones of the central chemoreceptors lie close to the respiratory centre and respond to changes in the hydrogen ion concentration in the cerebrospinal fluid (CSF). This is directly related to changes in blood carbon dioxide tension by the Henderson–Hasselbalch equation:

$$pH = pK + \log \frac{[HCO_3^-]}{0.003 P_{CO_2}}$$

An acute increase in carbon dioxide tension results in an increase in hydrogen ion concentration (a fall in pH), producing a reflex increase in ventilation. The blood–brain barrier is permeable to carbon dioxide but not to hydrogen ions.

The central chemoreceptors do not respond to changes in oxygen tension. Two groups of peripheral chemoreceptors are responsible for monitoring and responding to reductions in P_{aO_2}. The most important of these are the carotid bodies located at the bifurcation of the carotid arteries. The second group of arterial chemoreceptors are the aortic bodies located near the arch of the aorta. Although they do respond to changes in P_{CO_2} and hydrogen ion concentration, their primary function is the body's defence against hypoxia. Indeed, they are almost exclusively responsible for the ventilatory response to hypoxia in humans. There is a low level of activity in the carotid chemoreceptor nerves even at normal P_{aO_2}, and this increases only slightly with moderate hypoxia. The nerve discharge rate increases markedly, however, once P_{aO_2} falls below about 12 kPa. Maximum activity is reached when P_{aO_2} is approximately 2–3 kPa. Beyond this level, activity decreases, presumably due to the effects of the severe hypoxia on the sensory mechanisms.

NON-RESPIRATORY FUNCTIONS OF THE LUNGS

Because the entire blood volume passes through the lungs, they have a special role as a filter as well as some metabolic functions. The filtering function prevents particles from entering the arterial circulation, where the coronary and cerebral arteries are specifically vulnerable. The lungs also possess a well-developed proteolytic system, allowing thrombi to be cleared more rapidly from the lungs than from other organs.

The lung is a major extrahepatic site of the cytochrome P450 enzyme system, which is involved in the biotransformation of many drugs and xenobiotics. The lung plays a major role in the processing of hormones and vasoactive compounds. About 30% of circulating noradrenaline is taken up by the endothelium and inactivated. Serotonin (5-hydroxytryptamine) is almost completely removed from the circulation in the lung, and pulmonary clearance prevents recirculation. The lung is also a major site for the conversion of angiotensin I into angiotensin II by angiotensin-converting enzyme (ACE), present in abundance on the vascular surface of the pulmonary endothelium. The lung is also actively involved in the synthesis and metabolism of prostaglandins and thromboxanes.

Neutrophils and macrophages in the lung are involved in the formation of oxygen-derived free radicals for the killing of bacteria. Discharge of free radicals into the pulmonary circulation, thereby damaging the endothelium, causes capillary leak and may contribute to adult (acute) respiratory distress syndrome. Mast cells in the lung are a major source of histamine.

3

Neuromuscular physiology

Claude Meistelman, François Donati

INTRODUCTION

Neuromuscular transmission occurs through the release of acetylcholine at the motor endplate by motor neurones leading to the muscular contraction process. Both nerve and muscle cells can generate action potentials. Action potential, however, cannot propagate across the neuromuscular junction: transmission from nerve to muscle occurs through the medium of acetylcholine which is released into the synaptic cleft when the action potential reaches the nerve terminal. Acetylcholine binds to nicotinic acetylcholine receptors at the endplate, and causes the ion channel of the receptor to open. This makes the membrane potential less negative, that is a depolarisation occurs. When depolarisation reaches the threshold voltage, a muscle action potential is initiated, leading to muscular contraction

NEUROMUSCULAR JUNCTION

Each motor neurone runs as a large myelinated axon without interruption from the anterior horn of the grey matter in the spinal cord to the neuromuscular junction. A single axon innervates many muscle fibres. With a few exceptions (extraocular muscles and the upper oesophagus), human muscle cells are each innervated by a single axon. The axon, together with the muscle fibres that it innervates, is called a motor unit. The number of muscular fibres innervated by a single neurone ranges from 3 to 1000,

depending on the muscular function. Small muscles that react rapidly and whose control must be exact, such as the extraocular muscles and the muscles controlling the fingers, have few muscles in each motor unit. In contrast, large muscles that do not require fine control, such as the gastrocnemius, may have several hundred muscle fibres in their motor units.

A terminal branch of an axon approaches a specialised area of muscle, called the endplate, from which it is separated by a narrow gap, about 50 nm, called the synaptic cleft. Close to its terminal, the axon loses its myelin sheath. Schwann cells cover the whole nerve terminal area and, together with a basement membrane and protein filaments in the synaptic cleft, provide mechanical stability. The basement membrane contains some of the junctional acetylcholinesterase molecules. The muscle surface exhibits primary and secondary invaginations (Figure 3.1). The crests of these folds have a high density of nicotinic cholinergic receptors ($10\,000$–$20\,000/\mu m^2$). The troughs of the folds have a high density of sodium channels, which play a role in action potential propagation. The length of a neuromuscular junction varies from 20 to $50\,\mu m$ and depends on the diameter of the muscle fibre.[1] Most adult human muscles have a single endplate. The perijunctional zone contains a high density of sodium channels and a few cholinergic receptors in order to respond to endplate potentials.

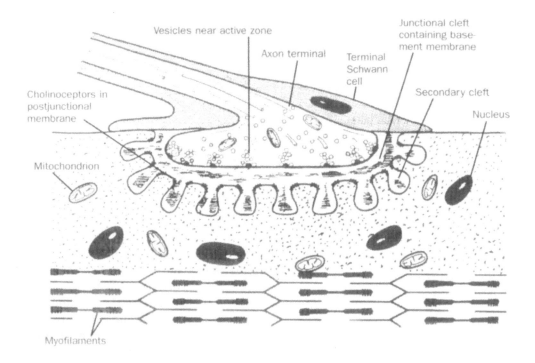

Figure 3.1 *General arrangement of a neuromuscular junction. From Bowman W.* Pharmacology of Neuromuscular Function, *2nd edn. London: Wright, 1990.*

NERVE ACTION POTENTIAL

Nerve and muscle cell interiors contain more potassium (K^+) than sodium (Na^+) ions, while the extracellular environment is rich in sodium. At rest, the membrane is more permeable to K^+ than Na^+, and this allows K^+ to flow out. The excess of positive ions on the outside creates a potential difference across the membrane, the inside of the cell being negative (-70 to -90 mV). A nerve action potential is a self-propagating wave of reversed membrane potential that passes along a nerve; it is usually triggered by the central nervous system. When the potential inside an excitable cell is made less negative (-15 mV) than the resting value, it activates a voltage-sensitive gated channel that is specific for sodium, and an inward sodium current is set up. During the rising phase of the action potential, the sodium conductance exceeds the potassium conductance and the net inward current drives the membrane potential to its peak; then the sodium conductance declines and the outward potassium current exceeds the inward sodium current, and the membrane potential to return to its resting value.

The purified sodium channel from mammalian tissues consists of a single large polypeptide α subunit of approximately 260 kD associated with two smaller β_1 and β_2 subunits of 36 and 33 kD respectively. The α and β_1 subunits extend across the membrane, whereas the β_2 subunit is linked to the α subunit by disulphide bonds and is apparently only exposed on the extracellular surface. The channel pore is formed only by the α subunit, the β subunits playing a role in the kinetics of channel opening and closing.

The action potential terminates by inactivation of sodium channels and activation of potassium channels. Both tend to bring the cell potential back to its resting value. In myelinated fibres, the sodium influx occurs only at the nodes of Ranvier, which are short gaps of unmyelinated axon separated by longer internodal myelinated regions where passive transmission occurs. These myelin segments are about 1 mm in length, while the nodes of Ranvier are only about 10 μm. Gated potassium channels are absent from mammalian nodes of Ranvier, so that the falling phase of the action potential is due to rapid inactivation of the sodium channels. Nerve action potentials last less than 1 ms. In large human myelinated fibres, which innervate skeletal muscles, the conduction velocity reaches 120 m/s. The puffer fish toxin tetrodotoxin acts from the extracellular side of the membrane to prevent the transition of the sodium channel to the open state. The main effect of tetrodotoxin is to block the conduction of action potentials without altering the resting membrane potential.

It is likely that active propagation of the action potential stops at the last node of Ranvier and electric activity reaches the nerve terminal by decremental spread. This allows the entry of calcium into the nerve through voltage-gated calcium channels, which causes further depolarisation. Voltage-gated potassium channels present in the non-myelinated terminals of the axons restore the cell potential to the resting value. 4-Aminopyridine increases the action potential duration and the inward calcium current by blocking potassium channels that hasten repolarisation.

SYNTHESIS AND STORAGE OF ACETYLCHOLINE

Acetylcholine is synthesised in the terminal axoplasm from choline and acetyl coenzyme A under the influence of the enzyme choline O-acetyltransferase before being stored in the nerve ending. Choline enters the axoplasm from the extracellular fluid by a sodium-dependent, high-affinity mechanism present in the membrane of cholinergic nerve endings. This is probably the rate-limiting step in the synthesis of acetylcholine. Approximately half of the choline produced by hydrolysis of acetylcholine by extracellular acetylcholinesterase is taken up and reused in the synthesis of new transmitter. Acetate is synthesised in the mitochondria from

pyruvate in the axon ending before combining with coenzyme A in the axoplasm.

Acetylcholine is present throughout the axoplasm, but its concentration is considerably higher in the nerve endings. After synthesis in the axoplasm, it is transported into synaptic vesicles, with an external diameter of about 45 nm. Between 50% and 80% of acetylcholine present in the nerve terminal is loaded actively in small vesicles that are manufactured by the Golgi apparatus before being loaded with acetylcholine, emptied, refilled, and reused. A large number of vesicles are concentrated near the cell membrane opposite the crests of the junctional folds of the endplate. Each vesicle contains approximately 10 000–12 000 molecules of acetylcholine. Transport of acetylcholine into the vesicles is mediated by a specific carrier protein. Energy for transport comes from an electrochemical proton gradient generated by the vesicular membrane V-type proton pumping ATPase. The second stage of the process involves exchange of intravesicular protons for cytoplasmic acetylcholine.[2] The loading process is inhibited by vesamicol, which inhibits the acetylcholine transporter.

RELEASE OF ACETYLCHOLINE

The vesicles tend to congregate close to the membrane and appear to form bands oriented parallel to the crests of the folds of the endplate, where the acetylcholine receptors lie. Only a small fraction of vesicles (1%) docked at the thickened part of the membrane (active zone) are immediately available for release. Recently synthesised acetylcholine is preferentially loaded in the immediately available store.[1] Vesicles of the reserve store are not free in the axoplasm, but are anchored to the actin strands and the microtubule cytoskeleton. Mobilisation of the reserve store occurs only when nerve activity becomes high. Synapsin I is a phosphorylated protein found in nerve terminals. Its role is to attach synaptic vesicles to elements of the cytoskeleton such as filaments of actin and to prevent vesicles from moving to the cell membrane. Synapsin I contains a binding site for a synaptic vesicle-associated calcium/calmodulin-dependent protein kinase II. Phosphorylation of synapsin by this kinase decreases the binding affinity of synapsin I to actin and synaptic vesicles, frees the synaptic vesicle from the synapsin, and facilitates the release of acetylcholine.

Synaptotagmin, synaptophysins, and synaptobrevin are integral vesicular membrane proteins involved in the docking of the vesicles at release sites and the formation of the fusion pore (Figure 3.2). Synaptotagmin, a vesicular membrane protein, binds to intracellular calcium. This induces a conformational change causing fusion of the immediately available vesicles with docking proteins that allow release of the vesicle content (acetylcholine, ATP, and calcium) into the synaptic cleft. Other vesicular membrane proteins such as synaptophysins and synaptobrevin are involved in acetylcholine release. Synaptophysin is one of the most abundant membrane proteins in synaptic vesicles. It may have a role in the binding of vesicles in the cytoskeleton and in transmitter release. Synaptobrevin is the site of action of botulinium toxin.

Acetylcholine is continuously and spontaneously released from the nerve endings in the absence of nerve impulses. This phenomenon induces small changes in the endplate resting potential. These miniature endplate potentials (MEPP) are uniform in magnitude (0.5–1 mV) and duration (a few milliseconds). They occur randomly at an average frequency of about 1 per second and are abolished by curare. An MEPP is due to the release of one quantum of acetylcholine, probably representing the contents of one vesicle. The MEPP is too small to produce a contraction because it does not bring the endplate potential to the threshold required to generate an action potential. When an action potential reaches the nerve terminal, approximately 200 quanta (~ 1–2 million acetylcholine vesicles) are simultaneously released and produce the full-size endplate potential (EPP), which triggers the chain of events leading to muscle contraction. Release is dependent on intracellular calcium. Depolarisation of the nerve terminal causes the opening of voltage-dependent calcium channels and an inward calcium current.

POSTJUNCTIONAL RECEPTORS

The nicotinic receptors at the neuromuscular junction belong to a superfamily of ligand-gated receptors, which also includes glycine, gamma aminobutyric acid ($GABA_A$ and $GABA_C$) receptors, and 5-HT_3 serotonin receptors,[3] that incorporate an ion channel as part of their structure. The nicotinic receptors have five protein subunits, two α and one β, ε and δ subunits (Figure 3.3). In some types of the receptor the ε subunit is replaced by a γ subunit. The α subunits contain two adjacent cysteine molecules that are essential for acetylcholine binding. Each subunit has four membrane-spanning domains, M1, M2, M3 and M4 (Figure 3.4). The M2 and the N-terminal third of M1 transmembrane domains of each subunit contribute to the lining of the central ion channel.[4] An additional protein, rapsyn, is associated with the cytoplasmic side of the receptor. It is distinct from and weakly bound to the β subunit. Rapsyn links the receptor to the cytoskeleton and contributes to the normal tight packing of nicotinic receptors at the crests of folds in the postsynaptic membrane. The number of receptors per endplate is of the order of 10^7.

Muscle nicotinic receptors fall into two main classes: mature (or adult) and immature (or fetal) (Figure 3.5). The immature (formerly called the extrajunctional) receptor has a γ instead of an ε subunit. It is found in fetal muscle prior to innervation before being replaced by mature receptors, and then disappears almost completely. Normal receptors at the neuromuscular junction are of the mature type. Immature receptors are found in relatively small numbers in extrajunctional locations on the membrane of normal skeletal muscles. Denervation causes these receptors to proliferate. Prolonged block of mature receptors at the neuromuscular junction also increases the number of immature receptors and causes terminal sprouting. Immature receptors have increased sensitivity to acetylcholine and succinylcholine but decreased sensitivity to non-depolarising muscle relaxants compared

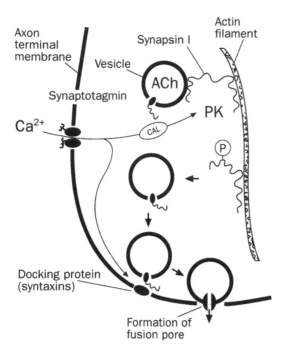

Figure 3.2 *Postulated mechanisms of the storage and release of acetylcholine. From Bowman W. Intensive Care Med 1993; **19** (Suppl 2): S45–53.*

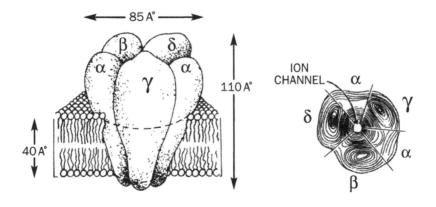

Figure 3.3 *Structure of the nicotinic acetylcholine receptor. From Taylor P. Anesthesiology 1985; **63**: 1–3.*

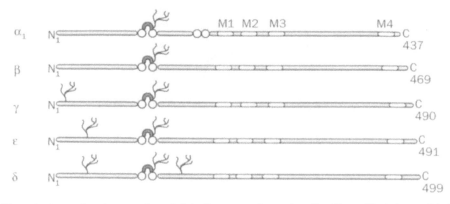

Figure 3.4 *Homologous structures of acetylcholine receptor subunits. From Lindstrom JM. Muscle Nerve 2000;* **23**: *453–77.*

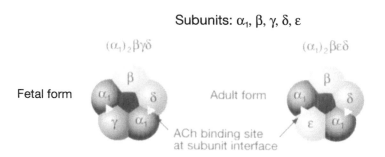

Subunits: α_1, β, γ, δ, ε

Figure 3.5 *Nicotinic acetylcholine (ACh) receptor subtypes. From Lindstrom JM. Muscle Nerve 2000;* **23**: *453–77.*

with mature receptors.[5] Their lifetimes are about 20 h whereas the lifetimes of mature receptors are many days or weeks.

The two α subunits each carry a single recognition site for nicotinic agonists such as acetylcholine and also for antagonists such as curare or α-bungarotoxin. The two recognition sites differ in their ligand-binding properties, probably due to the contribution of the other subunits. Substituting the ε for a γ subunit changes the affinity for both agonists and antagonists. Acetylcholine binds to the α subunit, probably at a site located between the 172nd and 201st amino acid from the N-terminal. This segment is located extracellularly, before the first transmembrane domain. When two acetylcholine molecules bind simultaneously to the pentameric complex, they induce a conformational change that opens the ion channel.

At rest, the receptor channel pore is closed. Occupation of both α subunits by an agonist such as acetylcholine induces a conformational change of the proteins that forms the pore. The size of the open channel (0.65 nm) is selective for small cations (Na^+, K^+, and Ca^{2+}). The ion channel appears to be composed of two distinct structural domains: an upper 'α-helical component' that delimits both the wide portion of the pore and the pharmacological site for non-competitive antagonists, and a lower 'loop component' that contributes to the narrowest part of the channel and to its selectivity.[6] During a mean channel open time of about 1 ms in the frog, approximately 10^4 ions flow through the channel. Only cations are able to flow through the channel, but there is little selectivity among different cations. When the muscle cell membrane is at its resting potential, the net driving force for potassium is near zero because the electrical gradient puts a brake on the outward movement of potassium ions. For sodium, both the concentration and the voltage gradients act in the same direction to drive the ion into the cell. The same is true for calcium, but its extracellular concentration is much lower than that of sodium. Therefore, during the opening of the mature nicotinic receptor channel, as many as 10 000 sodium ions might be allowed to pass through. The open time of the channel is agonist- and receptor-dependent. Acetylcholine dissociates from the receptor in a much shorter time than the mean duration of opening (1 ms). Immature receptors have a longer open time (6 ms), which could partly explain the hyperkalaemia after succinylcholine administration observed in patients with denervation.

Once released from the neurone, acetylcholine is subject to hydrolysis by acetylcholinesterase. About 80% of the acetylcholine molecules released might escape hydrolysis and bind to the nicotinic receptors. Almost all of these molecules are broken down after they dissociate from the receptors. The efficiency of the system is enhanced by the close proximity of the areas of release, called active zones, to the crests of the folds, where receptors are densely packed. The EPP is the consequence of the activation and simultaneous opening of several hundred thousand channels which causes a massive inward current of sodium ions and depolarises the membrane.[1] The EPP is not propagated but simply declines with distance from the endplate and time.

When the EPP reaches the excitation threshold (-50 to -40 mV), an action potential is initiated in the muscle by voltage-gated sodium channels. The action potential behaves like an all-or-nothing phenomenon that passes around the sarcolemma to activate the contractile mechanism. The sodium channel involved in the action potential is, like the nicotinic receptor, a protein structure shaped like a doughnut lying across the full thickness of the cell membrane. Unlike the nicotinic receptor, the doughnut is made up of a single α subunit. Two smaller units (β_1 and β_2) lie in the external half of the membrane. The sodium channel goes from a closed to an open position when the muscle membrane is depolarised by the endplate potential. It responds only to electrical changes and cannot be activated by agonists. At the peak of the action potential, the sodium channels inactivate. Activation of potassium channels then tends to restore the membrane potential towards its resting value.

The endplate and the surrounding area, called the perijunctional area, are rich in sodium channels, which, unlike nicotinic receptors, only allow inward movement of sodium ions. When the electrical potential inside the cell becomes more positive, a positive feedback occurs and sodium channels open in response to depolarisation. This phenomenon produces more depolarisation, which in turn cause more sodium channels to open.

PREJUNCTIONAL RECEPTORS

There is evidence for the presence of nicotinic acetylcholine receptors on motor nerve endings. Their presence has been suggested by the observations of fade after train-of-four or tetanic stimulation during non-depolarising neuromuscular block. Experiments have demonstrated that small concentrations of many agonists (including acetylcholine, nicotine, and carbachol) increase the evoked release of acetylcholine. This evoked release is prevented by curare and other related nicotinic antagonists. It is supposed that some of the released acetylcholine acts via a feedback mechanism on the nerve endings to simulate mobilisation of acetylcholine and increase its release at the synapse. The net effect of this positive feedback via presynaptic receptors is to sustain acetylcholine mobilisation in the face of continuing stimulation. These prejunctional receptors are likely of a different type than postjunctional receptors, and are not blocked by α-bungarotoxin. The presence of nicotinic receptors containing α_3 subunits, with a relatively high selectivity for calcium, has been demonstrated at motor nerve endings. They appear to be coupled to specific voltage-gated calcium channels that act through synaptotagmin and synapsin I to enhance vesicular fusions and to mobilise vesicles into the immediately available store.[7]

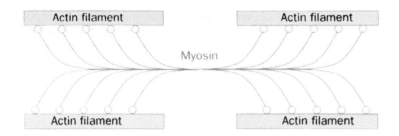

Figure 3.6 *Arrangement of cross-bridges between the heads of myosin and actin filaments in striated muscle.*

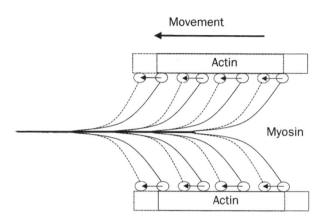

Figure 3.7 *An illustration of the 'sliding filament' theory of muscle contraction. Muscle contraction involves filaments of myosin and actin sliding over each other. This motion is produced by the myosin head attaching to active sites on the actin molecule, pulling the latter over the myosin molecule. The attachment is then broken and the head makes a new attachment for the next movement cycle.*

SKELETAL MUSCLE CONTRACTION

Muscle cells are multinucleated elongated cells containing myofilaments that slide over each other. These myofilaments are of two types: thick filaments composed of the protein myosin and thin filaments composed mainly of the protein actin but with a complex of two other proteins, troponin and tropomyosin. The striated appearance of muscle under the microscope is produced by the interdigitation of the thick myosin and the thinner actin filaments. Myofilaments are grouped into larger longitudinal structures called myofibrils. The sarcoplasmic reticulum is a membrane-bound structure that acts as a specialised reservoir for calcium ions. In most mammalian muscle fibres, it runs parallel to the myofibrils.

The action potential activates the contractile mechanism via the T tubules (invaginations of the cell membrane into the cytoplasm), the contractile proteins, and the sarcoplasmic reticulum. During normal transmission, the action potential is generated at the endplate and spreads simultaneously to both ends of the muscle fibre. The conduction velocity of this electrical impulse is slower in muscle (5–10 m/s) than in nerve (50–100 m/s). The spread of the action potential throughout the muscle fibre causes opening of voltage-gated calcium channels and a sudden influx of calcium, which is normally sequestrated in the sarcoplasmic reticulum. Calcium binds to troponin, and this removes the inhibitory effect of troponin on actin and myosin. The process of contraction is a consequence of cross-bridges between the globular heads of myosin filaments and the G-actin units of the thin filaments (Figure 3.6). In a poorly understood mechanism, the myosin heads undergo a conformational change, in the process pulling the actin filaments towards the centre of the myofibril in a ratchet-like mechanism (Figure 3.7). This is the 'sliding filament theory' of muscle contraction. Restoration of the relaxed state requires that calcium be removed from the troponine–tropomyosin complex, which can re-exert its inhibitory action on cross-bridge formation.[1] A new cycle of cross-bridge formation and detachment can now take place. Reuptake of calcium into the sarcoplasmic reticulum is active and requires energy.

The duration of the action potential is only a few milliseconds, after which there is a delay before contraction starts. The time course of a muscle contraction is much longer: it is approximately 100–200 ms. The twitch tension plotted against time has a rapid upstroke followed by a slower relaxation phase. If a nerve is stimulated at a relatively high frequency (>10 Hz), the muscle does not have time to relax between stimulations and fusion of contractions, a tetanus, occurs. The net result is a force of contraction greater than that associated with a single twitch.

Neuromuscular blocking agents do not affect excitation–contraction coupling, because they decrease both the electrical and mechanical events proportionally. In contrast, dantrolene acts at a stage after action potential propagation, which remains unaltered. It affects excitation–contraction coupling by inhibiting the release of calcium from the sarcoplasmic reticulum into the sarcoplasm and impairing the formation of cross-bridges.

MUSCLE TYPES

Muscles can be classified into several categories. Those with tonic or slow fibres, very common in non-mammalian vertebrates, are characterized by the existence of more than one endplate, the absence of a propagated action potential, and the production of a slow, graded, sustained contraction. This type of muscle is rare in humans and is probably restricted to extraocular muscles, intrinsic laryngeal muscles, and striated muscles in the upper oesophagus and the middle ear.

With few exceptions, mammalian muscles are composed almost entirely of focally innervated twitch fibres that can propagate an action potential and respond in an all-or-nothing fashion with a rapid contraction. They can be classified into three main subtypes according to their morphological, biochemical, and functional characteristics. Type I (slow red) have low contraction and relaxation speeds, and contain more sarcoplasmic reticulum than other fibres. Type IIA (fast red) combine fast contraction speed and resistance to fatigue. Type IIB (fast pale) have lit-

tle sarcoplasmic reticulum, and a high contraction speed. They are not suited for sustained work. The speed of contraction depends on the proportion of fibre types. The adductor pollicis is predominantly made up of type I fibres whereas the respiratory muscles contain an approximately equal mixture of type I and II fibres.

ACTION OF MUSCLE RELAXANTS

Non-depolarising muscle relaxants (NDMRs) bind competitively to the same site as acetylcholine on the α subunit of the nicotinic postjunctional receptor. Binding of one nicotinic antagonist molecule to one of the two α subunits of the receptor prevents opening of the channel because both α subunits need to be bound by acetylcholine for activation of the channel. In a given situation, the proportion of receptors bound to the agonist depends on the affinity of the binding site for the agonist, on its affinity for the antagonist and on the concentrations of agonist and antagonist. There is a considerable excess of acetylcholine released by a nerve impulse over that required to evoke the critical magnitude of endplate potential necessary to reach the threshold for a propagating action potential.[1] Only a small fraction of receptors need to bind acetylcholine to produce depolarisation. This has been referred as the margin of safety' of neuromuscular transmission. Non-depolarising neuromuscular block is not apparent until a large number of receptors are occupied by the muscle relaxant. About 75% of receptors must be occupied by a NDMR before a decrease in twitch height becomes apparent. Block is usually complete in peripheral muscles when 92% of receptors are occupied. Peripheral muscles have a smaller margin of safety than the diaphragm. The high margin of safety of respiratory muscles ensures that synaptic transmission is protected against moderate changes in quantal contents, which can occur when the nerve is stimulated at high frequency.

The block produced by an NDMR is not preceded by muscle fasciculations and is characterized by fade to repetitive stimulation and tetanus. Following tetanic stimulation, synthesis of acetylcholine is increased, which continues for some time after cessation of stimulation. This results in post-tetanic facilitation where a muscle response to a single stimulus or TOF is enhanced. NDMRs can also block the open receptor because they can have access to the mouth of the open channel but cannot pass through, thus preventing further ionic movement. This type of block is non-competitive and its role is probably marginal.

Succinylcholine produces a depolarisation of the postsynaptic membrane that is similar to but more persistent than that achieved by acetylcholine. The onset of neuromuscular block is characterized by an excitatory state with fasciculations of muscle fibres, thought to represent random repetitive neuronal firing. It could also be due to depolarisation of prejunctional receptors, and abolition of fasciculations by *d*-tubocurarine may represent action at the these receptors. The neuromuscular block by succinylcholine is characterized by a twitch response to indirect stimulation, which is diminished, but sustained with repetitive stimulation (i.e. absence of fade). It is associated with endplate depolarisation and the development of a surrounding zone of inexcitability through which a muscle action potential evoked by direct stimulation cannot propagate. An endplate potential evoked by nerve stimulation cannot excite the muscle fibre as a whole because the surrounding zone of inexcitability prevents the propagation of action potentials to the normally polarised muscle fibre membrane.[8] During prolonged depolarisation, the muscle may gain sodium and chloride and lose significant amounts of potassium – sufficient to raise serum levels of this ion. With continuous administration, a 'phase II block' develops, characterized by fade and post-tetanic facilitation. One of the mechanisms for this could be excessive activation of presynaptic nicotinic receptors, leading to reduced transmitter output. It could also be due to desensitisation of the endplate, which then becomes refractory to chemical stimulation.

The action of NDMRs is reversed by anticholinesterase drugs, which temporarily inactive acetylcholinesterase and increase the amount of acetylcholine at the postsynaptic membrane. They are not true antagonists because their action is mainly by increasing the amount of acetylcholine at the endplate. Edrophonium binds with the esteratic site on acetylcholinesterase, forming a loose electrostatic bond. The action is terminated by simple diffusion from the synaptic cleft. Neostigmine binds more strongly to both the anionic and esteratic sites on acetylcholinesterase. Like acetylcholine, neostigmine is hydrolysed by acetylcholinesterase, but the hydrolysis is extremely slow compared with that of acetylcholine and hence acetylcholinesterase is inhibited. The mechanism of action of anticholinesterase drugs has another consequence, namely a ceiling effect. Thus, increasing the dose beyond a certain point does not increase their ability to reverse the blocking effects of NDMRs.

REFERENCES

1. Bowman WC. *Pharmacology of neuromuscular function*. London: Butterworth & Co., 1990.
2. Sudhof TC, Jahn R. Proteins of synaptic vesicles involved in exocytosis and membrane recycling. *Neuron* 1991; **6**: 665–77.
3. Benfenati F, Valtorta F, Rubenstein JL, et al. Synaptic vesicle-associated Ca^{2+}/calmodulin-dependent protein kinase II is a binding protein for synapsin I. *Nature* 1992; **359**: 417–20.
4. Zhang H, Karlin A. Contribution of the beta subunit M2 segment to the ion-conducting pathway of the acetylcholine receptor. *Biochemistry* 1998; **37**: 7952–64.
5. Martyn JA, White DA, Gronert GA, et al. Up-and-down regulation of skeletal muscle acetylcholine receptors. Effects on neuromuscular blockers. *Anesthesiology* 1992; **76**: 822–43.
6. Corringer PJ, Le Novere N, Changeux JP. Nicotinic receptors at the amino acid level. *Annu Rev Pharmacol Toxicol* 2000; **40**: 431–58.
7. Bowman WC. Physiology and pharmacology of neuromuscular transmission, with special reference to the possible consequences of prolonged blockade. Intensive Care Med. 1993; **19** Suppl 2:S45-53.
8. Meistelman C, McLoughlin C. Suxamethonium – current controversies. *Curr Anaesthesia Crit Care* 1993; **4**: 53–8.

4

Gastrointestinal physiology

Cormac C McLoughlin

INTRODUCTION

The gastrointestinal tract has two major functions: processing of ingested food with a view to providing nourishment for the body and excretion of indigestible items from food and biliary secretion. These apparently simple tasks pose very significant problems:

- *The challenge of maintaining forward propulsive movement of food ingested intermittently without overstressing any part of the intestine.* This requires a storage organ (stomach), one-way valves (sphincters) to maintain controlled propulsive movement, and a complex interplay of neural and hormonal influences to control general and regional motility.
- *A variety of secretions to break down the various chemical components of food.* As the conditions required for this are hostile to the body and the enzymes are potentially damaging to body tissues, protective barriers to prevent autodigestion and mechanisms for controlling secretion are required. This again is dependent on a number of neural and hormonal influences with stimulatory and inhibitory actions.
- *Digestion of fat, carbohydrate, and protein to produce component molecules.* This requires thorough mixing with digestive juices, and, despite difficulties with solubility (particularly with fat), must be accomplished within a fairly short period of time.

- *Absorption of various chemical compounds and their processing into an appropriate condition for transport into the body.* This requires an enormous surface area for absorption and both active and passive transport systems.

All of these activities must occur in concert and with minimal waste of bodily resources such as fluid and protein.

GENERAL DESCRIPTION

The gastrointestinal tract is composed of the mouth, oesophagus, stomach, and the small and large intestines, altogether about 4.5 m in length. Accessory structures are the salivary glands, pancreas, liver, and gallbladder. Total daily secretion in an adult amounts to about 7 l, most of which is reabsorbed, leaving a daily loss in faeces of about 100 ml. Blood flow is through the splanchnic circulation, which takes about 25% of the cardiac output and drains via the portal vein to the liver. The portal circulation begins and ends in capillaries and contributes about two-thirds of the total liver blood flow. The wall of the digestive tract contains smooth muscle, except for the upper third of the oesophagus and the external anal sphincter with skeletal muscle, which gives conditioned voluntary control. Although digestive secretions enter the lumen from the stomach and liver, the principal organ for digestion of protein, carbohydrate, and fat is the pancreas.

Smooth muscle in different sections of the intestinal tract has different basic electrical rhythms, expressed as different patterns of motility. An important characteristic of gastrointestinal motility is that contractile function is further influenced by short reflexes mediated by intrinsic myenteric nerve plexus activity and long reflexes relayed via vagus and sympathetic nerves. Local and systemic activity of intestinal peptides such as gastrin and secretin influence motility and release of digestive secretions. Propulsive activity is achieved by *phasic contractions* with rolling segmental contractions (segmentation), which improves mixing of food and digestive enzymes and contact with absorptive epithelium, and with peristalsis, a slow contractile movement over short distances. In contrast, sphincters are often maintained in tonic contraction over several hours, relaxing in response to approaching waves of contraction.

SWALLOWING

The oesophagus transmits food from the pharynx to the stomach. Negative pressure transmitted from the pleural cavities produces a pressure in the lumen of the thoracic oesophagus that is lower than those in the pharynx and the stomach. Tendency to draw in contents from the stomach or air from the pharynx is prevented by closure of the upper and lower oesophageal sphincters. Reflux of food due to the higher pressures in the stomach is further prevented by the subdiaphragmatic location of the terminal part of the oesophagus.

As a prelude to swallowing, solid food is chewed and mixed with saliva. Chewing breaks food up into manageable sizes for swallowing, and saliva lubricates the mouth and initiates, in a minor way, some digestion of starch. Saliva is produced in response to sight, smell, or taste of food and to the physical presence of food in the mouth. About 1–2 l/day are produced from the parotid, submaxillary, and sublingual glands. This consists of mucin from the sublingual and submandibular glands, and ptyalin or salivary amylase from the parotid and submandibular glands. Saliva is rich in bicarbonate and is slightly alkaline, which helps to neutralize the acid produced by oral bacteria. Uniquely, production of saliva is mediated by sympathetic and parasympathetic innervation, with the latter being the most important influence.

Swallowing is a complex reflex controlled by the swallowing centre in the medulla and requiring responses occurring in a timed sequence. It is initiated when food reaches the pharynx and is accompanied by a raising of the soft palate to close off the nasopharynx and an inhibition of respiration. The larynx is raised, the glottis is closed, and the upper oesophageal sphincter relaxes. Food is conducted to the stomach by peristalsis, each wave taking about 9 s to reach the stomach. Vagal efferents synapse with internal nerve plexuses and coordinate the progress of the peristaltic wave and relaxation of the lower oesophageal sphincter.

Gastric function

Food is generally presented to the stomach in small soft boluses, prepared in the mouth by chewing and moistened by saliva, containing mucins and ptyalin. As a result of its large capacity, the stomach is capable of accommodating a significant quantity of food without a large increase in intragastric pressure. Its main function is to maintain an environment where its digestive enzymes can commence protein digestion and to move food at a controlled rate via the pyloric sphincter into the duodenum. The major issues for gastric physiology are the nature and control of gastric secretion and the methods of controlling motility and gastric emptying. Not surprisingly, the system is integrated with considerable overlap in control of both functions.

Gastric secretion

Gastric secretion is of the order of 2–3 l/day from exocrine glands in the body and fundus of the stomach. There are three types of cells:

1. *Chief or peptic cells in the antrum, which secrete proteolytic proenzymes called pepsinogens.* To avoid cellular damage, they are inactive until

they enter the gastric lumen, where in the acid pH they are cleaved to form active pepsins that hydrolyse proteins.

2. *Parietal cells, which secrete hydrochloric acid and intrinsic factor.* The latter is important for the absorption of vitamin B_{12} in the terminal ileum. Hydrochloric acid secretion requires the production of H_2CO_3 in the cell interior, catalysed by carbonic anhydrase. The secretion of H^+ (Figure 4.1) is an active process involving a proton pump working against a 3 million-fold concentration gradient between the cell and gastric lumen and in which K^+ is exchanged. It produces a gastric pH of between 1 and 3, which kills bacteria, allows the activation of pepsin, and is optimum for its function (active at pH < 3.5). As acid secretion increases after eating, it is accompanied by an increase in pH of gastric venous blood (alkaline tide), with bicarbonate entering the blood in active exchange for chloride ion. This is mirrored, however, by bicarbonate secretion in pancreatic juices such that the body pH remains stable.

3. *Mucous cells, which secrete mucin.* This secretion is alkaline, has a protective role for mucosal cells, and may lubricate the gastric lumen. Inhibition of prostaglandin function disrupts mucin production, leaving gastric cells vulnerable to gastric acid.

Control of gastric acid secretion

There are three classical stages in the control of gastric secretion, which are mediated by short myenteric reflexes and long vagal reflexes and by systemic hormone secretion (Figure 4.2). More recently, the role of local peptides in modulating secretion and motility has become evident.

1. *The cephalic phase.* This refers to anticipatory secretion of HCl and pepsinogen in response to the smell, sight, or taste of food. This is mediated by acetylcholine from the vagus nerve, which acts via the internal nerve plexuses in the stomach wall to stimulate acid secretion. The same neural stimulus causes release of bombesin or gastrin-releasing peptide (GRP) from enteric neurones, which

stimulates so-called G cells within the antrum to release gastrin into the circulation. This hormone further stimulates parietal cells to secrete acid. Release of histamine from cells in gastric glands, which then binds to H_2 receptors on parietal cells, is thought to be a final common component of neural and hormonal stimulation of gastric acid secretion.

2. *The gastric phase.* This refers to the stage where the presence of food in the stomach produces gastric secretion. This arises from either gastric distension or the presence of food constituents. Polypeptides, in particular, cause direct stimulation of acid secretion and promote gastrin release, while G-cell activity is also promoted by gastric distension. An autoregulatory control also comes into play with acid inhibiting its own secretion by suppressing G-cell release of gastrin.

Acetylcholine via short and long neural reflexes in these first two phases is the major stimulus for pepsinogen secretion.

3. *The intestinal phase.* This represents the role of a number of feedback mechanisms to inhibit gastric secretion, and, as its name suggests, it originates in the duodenum. Stretching of the wall of the intestine, the presence of acid or digestive products, or hyperosmotic chyme causes a reduction of gastric secretion by gastrointestinal short and long nervous reflexes. Hormonal feedback is through the release of secretin and gastric inhibitory peptide (GIP) from mucosal cells in the small intestine. GIP also causes the release of somatostatin, which inhibits both parietal and G cells.

Gastric motility

When empty, the stomach takes part in slow peristaltic waves sweeping along the whole gastrointestinal tract at about 90-minute intervals. This is known as the migrating motor complex and is thought to be under the control of a candidate hormone, motilin. After eating, peristaltic waves run down the stomach from the fundus to the pylorus about three times per minute (basic electrical rhythm). Contraction of the pylorus

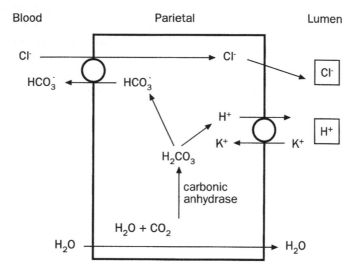

Figure 4.1 *Mechanism of gastric acid secretion with active secretion of H^+ ions, dependent on H^+/K^+-ATPase, from the parietal cell into the gastric lumen and Cl^- in exchange for HCO_3^- between parietal cell and blood*

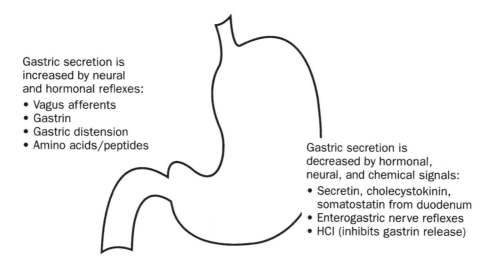

Gastric secretion is increased by neural and hormonal reflexes:
- Vagus afferents
- Gastrin
- Gastric distension
- Amino acids/peptides

Gastric secretion is decreased by hormonal, neural, and chemical signals:
- Secretin, cholecystokinin, somatostatin from duodenum
- Enterogastric nerve reflexes
- HCl (inhibits gastrin release)

Figure 4.2 *Stimulatory and inhibitory neural and hormonal influences in gastric secretion. Gastric acid autoregulates by the inhibition of gastrin release, while the presence of food in the duodenum gives rise to negative feedback mediated by long and short nervous reflexes and the release of hormones and messenger peptides.*

has important functions both by limiting exit of chyme into the duodenum and by promoting retropulsion of food into the body of the stomach to improve mixing of food and digestive juices. The strength of contraction and gastric emptying is determined by the interplay of stimulatory neural and hormonal influences originating within the stomach, and so-called enterogastric inhibitory reflexes mediated by neural and hormonal effects from the duodenum (Figure 4.3).

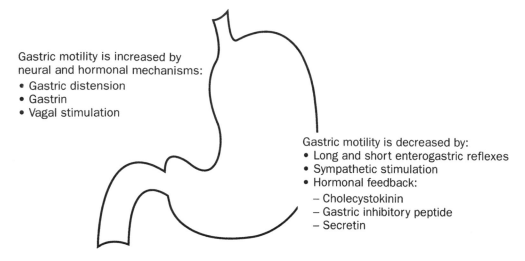

Gastric motility is increased by neural and hormonal mechanisms:
- Gastric distension
- Gastrin
- Vagal stimulation

Gastric motility is decreased by:
- Long and short enterogastric reflexes
- Sympathetic stimulation
- Hormonal feedback:
  - Cholecystokinin
  - Gastric inhibitory peptide
  - Secretin

Figure 4.3 *The interplay between hormonal and neural influences affecting gastric motility and emptying. Neural mechanisms are mediated by intrinsic myenteric plexuses and extrinsic autonomic nerves. Hormonal feedback from the duodenum due to fat content and acidic and hyperosmolar chyme is an important regulator of gastric emptying.*

Gastric distension, as we saw earlier, promotes gastrin release by short reflexes from the gastric nerve plexus and long reflexes via the vagal nerve, and this hormone increases the strength of gastric contractions. Vagal activity, in itself, similarly promotes contraction while sympathetic activity decreases the force of contraction. This may delay gastric emptying following trauma, with pain or intense emotional states when sympathetic stimulation is high.

The presence of foodstuff within the duodenum feeds back to limit gastric emptying so that the duodenum can be protected against overdistension and the effects of gastric acid. The presence of acid causes release of the hormone secretin, while fat promotes the release of GIP and cholecystokinin from the duodenal mucosa. These bloodborne hormones reduce gastric motility. Inhibitory neural reflexes stimulated by duodenal distension, high osmolarity, and the presence of food products and mediated directly via the myenteric plexus or indirectly by extrinsic nerve reflexes have a similar modulating effect. The net effect is that while liquids have a short transit time through the stomach, gastric emptying of food will be determined by a number of factors, including emotional factors and the nature of food constituents, with food high in fat having the longest transit.

The factors influencing gastric secretion and motility as presented are, by necessity, an oversimplification of what is an extremely complex process. The regulation of function of the gastrointestinal system is also dependent on a number of messenger peptides present in cells within the digestive tract (Table 4.1). Endocrine peptides released into the circulation, and including the aforementioned gastrin, secretin, GIP, and possibly motilin, are probably among the best understood. Somatostatin, a paracrine peptide present in the wall of the stomach and small intestine, may be transported by local circulation and inhibits gastric and pancreatic secretion and also reduces intestinal motility. Neural peptide messengers released from nerve terminals within internal nerve plexuses include vasoactive intestinal polypeptide (VIP), which is thought to inhibit gastric and intestinal motility and gastric secretion.

The small intestine – motility, secretion, and digestion

The small intestine runs from the duodenum to

Table 4.1 Neuroendocrine factors in gastrointestinal function

Factor	Location	Action
Gastrin	Antral G cells	Stimulates acid secretion
Secretin	Enterochromaffin cells in small intestine	Stimulates bicarbonate in pancreatic secretions; inhibits gastric secretion and emptying
Cholecystokinin	Enterochromaffin cells in small intestine	Stimulates gallbladder contraction and pancreatic secretion; inhibits gastric secretion and emptying
Bombesin	Enteric neurones	Stimulates gastrin and pancreatic secretion
Gastric inhibitory peptide	Enterochromaffin cells	Inhibits gastric acid secretion and emptying
Motilin	Enterochromaffin cells	Regulates migrating myoelectric complex
Somatostatin	Enterochromaffin cells Enteric neurones	Inhibits gastric and pancreatic secretion
Vasoactive intestinal polypeptide	Enteric neurones	Relaxes intestinal smooth muscle; stimulates intestinal secretions
Substance P	Enteric neurones	Stimulates motility and intestinal secretions
Acetylcholine	Vagus and enteric nerves	Stimulates gastrointestinal secretion and smooth muscle contractility

the ileocaecal valve and is the principal site for digestion and absorption of nutrients. Contractile waves facilitate digestion of food and bring it into close contact with the intestinal mucosa. The highly folded mucosa (valvulae conniventes), with fingerlike villi each further divided into microvilli, provides an enormous surface area for absorption. The presence of enzymes within the microvilli facilitates terminal digestion. Segmental contraction of the bowel occurs at a rate of about 12 contractions per minute in the duodenum and 8 per minute in the ileum. Peristaltic propulsion initiated by distension and mediated by local myenteric reflexes propels food by proximal contraction and distal relaxation. Extrinsic nerves mediate intestino-intestinal reflexes, where stretching in one area of the bowel inhibits contractions in the rest of the bowel. Autonomic control via the vagus nerve and spinal sympathetic neurones has opposite effects on intestinal motility. Motility is stimulated by vagal activity and inhibited by sympathetic stimulation. Inhibition of sympathetic innervation of the gut by epidural analge-sia is a suggested mechanism for the earlier return of intestinal motility following abdominal surgery when this form of pain relief is used.

The ileocaecal sphincter controls the movement of chyme from the ileum into the caecum, and, although it is normally closed, it relaxes when motor activity in the ileum is increased.

Digestive function

Digestive processes within the small intestine are carefully orchestrated. The most important organ for digestive secretion is the pancreas, which releases secretions rich in bicarbonate and enzymes in response to hormonal stimulation by secretin and cholecystokinin. As we saw earlier, the presence of acid within the duodenum causes secretion of secretin, which stimulates the acinar cells of the exocrine pancreas to secrete juice rich in bicarbonate. This helps to neutralise acid within the lumen of the duodenum, raising the pH to near neutrality for optimum digestion. The resulting retention of hydrogen ions offsets the potential alkalosis that accompanies gastric acid secretion in the alkaline tide.

Protein and fat products cause secretion of cholecystokinin which stimulates secretion of digestive enzymes in the pancreatic juice. These are capable of breaking down protein, fat, and carbohydrate. Proteolytic enzymes are stored and released as inactive precursors (zymogens), which are then converted to active enzymes by the enzyme enterokinase present in the luminal membrane of epithelium in the small intestine. Thus trypsinogen is converted to trypsin, chymotryposinogen to chymotrypsin, and procarboxypeptidase to carboxypeptidase.

The pancreas also secretes pancreatic lipase, which is the only enzyme in the intestine breaking down fat into monoglycerides and fatty acids. Pancreatic amylase, similar to salivary amylase, degrades starch, while ribonuclease and deoxribonuclease digest nucleic acids. An increase in pH and emptying of chyme from the duodenum removes the stimulus for release of secretin and cholecystokinin and thus controls pancreatic secretion. A total of about 1500 ml of pancreatic secretion is produced per day.

Biliary secretions, about 500 ml/day, are produced in the liver and diverted to the gallbladder between meals, when a closed sphincter of Oddi, at the lower end of the common bile duct, prevents bile from entering the duodenum. The principal constituents of bile are water, bicarbonate, bile pigments, cholesterol, and, most importantly, bile salts (cholate and chendeoxycholate). Contraction of the gallbladder and relaxation of the sphincter of Oddi to promote biliary flow occur in response to cholecystokinin.

Fat digestion is a major challenge for the intestine, as hydrophobic fat molecules form globules in an aqueous setting, leaving only a small surface area available for enzymatic degradation. Bile salts, however, allow the formation of a fat emulsion, thereby increasing the area of activity for pancreatic lipase. Additionally, bile salts interact with the monoglyceride and fatty acid products of fat metabolism to form very small aggregates called micelles, which are easily dispersed in solution for absorption.

Obstruction to bile flow impairs the absorption of dietary fat, including the fat-soluble vitamins A, D, E, and K.

Bile salts are reabsorbed by active transport in the distal ileum in an enterohepatic recirculation and recycled several times in one day. The control mechanism for bile production is through positive feedback of bile salt concentrations in the portal vein. High concentrations during a meal increases bile production.

Absorption

Water absorption is largely carried out in the small intestine, and is a passive process dependent on the active absorption of sodium and food products. Sodium is absorbed by an active transport system, and water follows by osmosis. The final digestion of protein and carbohydrates takes place in the microvilli of enterocytes (the intestinal brush border). Small peptides are broken down here by peptidases in the brush border and amino acids are then actively transported into the portal venous circulation. Digestible starches are broken down in the intestinal lumen to the disaccharides, maltose (two glucose molecules), lactose (glucose and galactose), and sucrose (glucose and fructose). The brush border contains maltase, lactase, and sucrase to complete digestion to monosaccharides. Transport of glucose and galactose into the portal circulation is by a carrier-mediated process coupled to the sodium pump. Fructose absorption occurs passively by facilitated diffusion.

Lipid absorption is more tortuous. Short-chain fatty acids are absorbed easily into the bloodstream. However, larger monoglyceride and long-chain fatty acid molecules are absorbed into the intestinal epithelium, where they are resynthesised into triglycerides and form droplets. Addition of a phospholipid and protein cover produces a chylomicron, which is extruded inwards and enters the central lacteal of the villus and is transported from there by lymphatic drainage to the systemic circulation.

The absorption of iron and calcium is adjusted to maintain body homeostasis. Specific calcium-binding proteins in the intestinal mucosa are regulated by vitamin D. Low serum levels of calcium stimulate an increase in 1,25-dihydroxy-cholecalciferol, which increases the amount of mucosal calcium-binding protein.

Absorption of iron is carefully controlled, as the ion in excess is toxic to body tissues and cannot easily be excreted once it has entered the circulation. About 10% of dietary iron is absorbed (more if iron stores are low). An active uptake process in the upper small intestine takes divalent (ferrous) iron (Fe^{2+}) into the luminal cells, where it combines with a cellular storage protein apoferritin to form ferritin. Apoferritin is available for further iron binding only when the iron plasma carrier protein transferrin is desaturated and available to take up iron from this cellular store.

The gastrointestinal tract has an extensive immune system. Mucosa-associated lymphoid tissue (MALT) includes the tonsils and adenoids and diffuse tissue throughout the gut. Peyer's patches are discrete collections of lymphoid cells in the intestine, containing T and B cells. Antigens in the intestine are sampled and stimulate production of T lymphocytes and B lymphocytes, the latter producing IgA immunoglobulin, which is concentrated in digestive secretions. This active protection against luminal pathogens is combined with a phenomenon known as oral tolerance, which prevents the immune system from responding to common luminal antigens. Failure to suppress this immune tolerance may be associated with some forms of inflammatory bowel disease.

The large intestine

The large intestine is just over 1 m in length and extends from the ileocaecal valve to the anus. While it does not contain villi or digestive enzymes, it does secrete an alkaline mucus rich in potassium and bicarbonate to protect the mucosa and lubricate the faeces. About 1500 ml of chyme per day enters the colon and all but about 100 ml of water is reabsorbed passively with active sodium reabsorption. Whereas there are few bacteria in the small intestine, the large intestine is rich in bacterial flora, which synthesise

a small amount of vitamins. These, however, are of little dietary significance.

The ileocaecal valve is usually closed, but, after eating, it opens with contraction in the distal ileum. Motility, both by segmentation and by peristalsis, occurs as in the small intestine but at a slower rate, while, after eating, an intense contraction is stimulated, which spreads rapidly over the colon to the rectum. This is attributed to a gastrocolic reflex.

Distension of the rectum elicits the desire to defecate and is accompanied by increased muscular activity in the sigmoid colon, contraction of the rectum, and relaxation of the internal and external anal sphincters. This defecation reflex is mediated by intrinsic myenteric nerves and extrinsic sacral spinal nerves. Voluntary control can override relaxation of the external sphincter, and defecation itself can be voluntarily augmented by raising intra-abdominal pressure on straining.

Nausea and vomiting

Nausea is an unpleasant subjective sensation of impending vomiting and is sometimes associated with epigastric discomfort. Vomiting is an active process under the control of the vomiting centre, and involves the active muscular expulsion of stomach contents in a reflex that, like swallowing, involves carefully timed respiratory and peristaltic responses. As an evolutionary development, it undoubtedly bestows advantages in both removal of harmful material from the body and discouragement of ingestion of toxic materials.

The vomiting centre lies in the dorsal part of the lateral reticular formation in the medulla oblongata of the brainstem. It receives inputs from a variety of sources, including the cerebral cortex, which can produce vomiting associated with emotion and unpleasant somatic sensations. The predominant receptor types are dopamine (D_2), serotonin (5-HT_3), and acetylcholine. The chemoreceptor trigger zone (CTZ) is located in what is known as the area postrema in the floor of the fourth ventricle and relays to the vomiting centre. It represents the major area of input into the vomiting centre. Lying outside the bloodbrain barrier, it is sensitive to chemical stimuli from drugs such as opioids and blood-borne toxins. The most prevalent receptor sub-types in the CTZ are dopamine, acetylcholine, and serotonin.

Motion, which causes endolymph movement within the inner ear, stimulates histamine (H_1) and muscarinic acetylcholine receptors in the vestibular apparatus, and this sends impulses to the CTZ via the eighth cranial nerve and vestibular nucleus. This gives rise to the nausea associated with inner ear pathology and travel sickness.

Vagal and sympathetic nerves carry impulses from viscera such as the mediastinum and intestinal tract, relaying to the vomiting centre via the nucleus tractus solitarius and CTZ. Intestinal receptors are sensitive to distension of the gut wall and also carry impulses from chemoreceptors in the upper small intestine. The latter are stimulated by irritants and hypertonic solutions, probably mediated by release of serotonin from enterochromaffin cells.

Nausea associated with surgery is multifactorial in origin, related to the site of surgery, the degree of handling of the bowel, the drugs used, and the predisposition of the patient. This is reflected in the success of combinations of antiemetic medications over single-therapy approach.

The act of vomiting, initiated by the vomiting centre, involves integration of respiratory, peristaltic and vascular reflexes involving a number of cranial nerves (5th, 9th, 10th, and 11th) and spinal nerves supplying the abdominal musculature. It is often preceded by pallor, increased heart rate, salivation, and sweating. A deep inspiration accompanies closure of the glottis and inhibition of further respiration. Descent of the diaphragm and repeated contraction of abdominal muscles raises intragastric pressure, and retrograde contractions of the stomach and small intestine force gastric contents into the oesophagus as the lower oesophageal sphincter relaxes. This retching manoeuvre precedes relaxation of the upper oesophageal sphincter, which allows food to be expelled in the act of vomiting.

When vomiting is prolonged or violent, it may have detrimental effects, including metabolic derangement (dehydration, metabolic acidosis, and loss of Na^+, K^+, Cl^-, and HCO_3^-), bleeding from under surgical flaps, wound dehiscence, and lower oesophageal tears (Mallory–Weiss).

FURTHER READING

American Physiological Society. *Handbook of Physiology.* Section 6: *The Gastrointestinal System.* Baltimore: Waverley Press, 1989.

Heuman DM, Mills AS, McGuire HH. *Gastro-enterology.* Philadelphia: WB Saunders, 1997.

5

Mechanisms of pain

William I Campbell

INTRODUCTION

The ability to illicit painful sensation is essential for the well-being of any organism, since its function is to prevent harm. Classic thinking proposed that a noxious stimulus travelled by a series of pathways to the brain, where the region of potential injury could be identified and if necessary withdrawn, by either voluntary or unconscious reflex action. It is now known that before a noxious sensation is elicited as pain it must be processed by higher centres within the central nervous system (CNS). A definition of pain that reflects this states that pain is 'an unpleasant sensory and emotional experience associated with actual or potential tissue damage or described in terms of such damage'. This definition takes into account the fact that emotional and evaluative processes come into play and that although tissue damage may not necessarily be taking place, the sensation may feel as such.

PERIPHERAL NOCICEPTION

The conduction of nociceptive information from the periphery to the CNS is carried out by neurones that have a bipolar structure. The tip of the peripheral axon lies within the appropriate tissue in which nociceptive information is to be detected. The cell body lies within the dorsal root ganglion (DRG), with the proximal axon running into the dorsal aspect of the spinal cord. Due to the uneven distribution of ions within and outside the cell membrane, the resting membrane potential of these cells is 50–100 mV, with the positive charge being on the outside of the cell. An adenosine triphosphatase (ATPase) pump continuously keeps the concentration of sodium outside the cell at 20 times of that within the cell. Conversely, this pumping system maintains a potassium concentration inside the cell at 35 times of that outside. When the neurone is activated, there is an influx of sodium into the cell, so that the outside charge becomes either neutral or negative. This results in an action potential, and it can only run in one direction due to the refractory phase that follows membrane depolarisation – in nociceptors that is from the periphery towards the spinal cord. There are two types of nociceptor: fast conducting Aδ fibres and the more slowly conducting C fibres.

Cutaneous Aδ fibres are myelinated with Schwann cell envelopes at 1.5 mm intervals throughout their length, the gaps between adjacent envelopes being called the nodes of Ranvier. This myelin sheath forms a hydrophobic lipoprotein barrier. The axon is approximately 3 μm in diameter and has a conduction velocity in the range of 12–30 m/s. This speed of axonal conduction is a function of the axonal diameter, but is facilitated due to the jumping of electrical activity between the nodes of Ranvier – salutatory conduction. This is important for the rapid transfer of information from the periphery to the spinal cord. These fibres are high-threshold receptors, which respond to mechanical stimulation, such as a firm pinch. Some of the fibres also respond to noxious heat (>45°C). Aδ-fibre activation results in a sharp, well-localised 'first pain'.

The C fibres do not have a myelin sheath and are approximately 1 μm in diameter. They conduct much more slowly than the Aδ fibres, with typical velocities of 0.5–2 m/s. These receptors are sensitive to chemical and thermal stimulation, and are frequently referred to as polymodal nociceptors. Approximately 50% of the C-fibre population is referred to as 'silent' since they are unresponsive until prior sensitisation by the chemical mediators of inflammation. Overall, the C-fibre population is responsible for 80% of the nociceptive primary afferents, and the perception of this information tends to be associated with poorly localised, aching, and occasionally burning pain – 'second pain' (Table 5.1).

When tissue injury occurs, potassium and kinins are released from the damaged cells. These stimulate the receptor directly, resulting in the release of neuropeptides, such as substance P (SP), from the receptor. This in turn causes the degranulation of adjacent mast cells, with the production of platelet-activating factor (PAF), which in turn releases serotonin from the platelets. Histamine is also released from the mast cells, starting an inflammatory reaction within the tissues, with vasodilatation, lowered pH, and the release of prostanoids such as leukotrienes and prostaglandins (PGs) (Figure 5.1). These prostanoids, together with SP itself, sensitise the nociceptor rather than stimulate it directly (Figure 5.2), lowering its threshold to stimulation.

Bradykinin activates a number of inflammatory mediators:

- tumour necrosis factor α (TNF-α) which in turn activates interleukin-6 (IL-6) and IL-8, which increase PGs and sympathetic activity (Table 5.2); IL-6 is released from monocytes, fibroblasts, and endothelium;
- IL-1, which stimulates the induction of inducible nitric oxide synthase (i-NOS) and cycloxygenase-2 (COX-2).

All of these mediators result in an inflammatory response and hyperalgesia. The inflammatory response can be blocked by the use of steroids or non-steroidal anti-inflammatory drugs (NSAIDs). However, there are two types of hyperalgesia:

- *Primary hyperalgesia* is mediated by the reduction in activation thresholds of nociceptors due to the above activity.
- *Secondary hyperalgesia* is due to central sensitisation within the spinal cord, when the dorsal horn becomes so hyperexcitable that low-threshold stimuli mediated by Aβ fibres is detected as painful and there is an augmentation of Aδ-fibre information (also see later). This secondary hyperalgesia extends beyond the area of the primary hyperalgesia. It does not respond to anti-inflammatory agents but can be prevented by neural blockade of the area with local anaesthetic, prior to tissue insult.

SPINAL PATHWAYS

Nociceptive information within the Aδ and C fibres arrives at the dorsal horn of the spinal cord via the lateral part of the dorsal root. The dorsal root ganglion contains the cell bodies of both types of nociceptor, together with other sensory neurones such as Aα and Aβ fibres. The latter two groups of fibres conduct information associated with muscle spindles and touch respectively. Most C fibres terminate in the superficial dorsal horn, at lamina II (also known as the substantia gelatinosa). Aδ fibres largely terminate in laminae I and V. Upon reaching the dorsal horn, all types of sensory fibre tend to branch, sending information in an ascending and descending fashion amongst several segments in Lissauer's tract, before penetrating the dorsal horn and synapsing with other neurones.

Aδ fibres terminate mainly in laminae I and V, with some of their high-threshold fibres ending directly in lamina II. Most cutaneous C fibres terminate in lamina II. However, visceral C fibres terminate at laminae I, II, IV, V, and X. The neurones at lamina I respond to high-intensity noxious stimulation, together with projection neurones, which respond to low threshold

Table 5.1 Different types of primary afferent fibre involved in nociception, together with their destinations in the laminae of Rexed

Fibre type	Diameter (μm)	Velocity (m/s)	Function	Destination
Aβ	6–17	30–75	Low threshold mechanoreceptors	Laminae II and IV
Aδ	1–5	5–30	High-threshold mechanoreceptors	Laminae I and V
C	0.3–1.5	0.5–2	Polymodal nociceptors	Lamina II

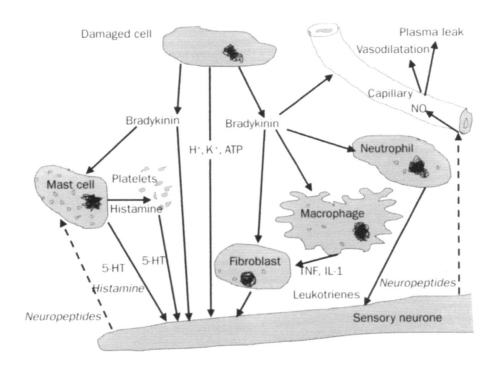

Figure 5.1 *The effects of inflammatory mediators released following cell damage to induce pain through the release of adenosine triphosphate (ATP), bradykinin, hydrogen (H⁺) and potassium (K⁺). Bradykinin also promotes the release of histamine and serotonin (5-HT) from mast cells, prostaglandins (PGs) from fibroblasts, and leukotrienes from neutrophils. These latter two agents sensitise the sensory neurone to the previous algesic substances. Neuropeptides such as substance P and glutamate are released from the neurone, perpetuating the inflammatory response. These also induce vasodilatation and plasma leakage from capillaries. See also Table 5.2 for the additional effects of these agents. (NO, nitric oxide; TNF, tumour necrosis factor; IL-1, interleukin-1.)*

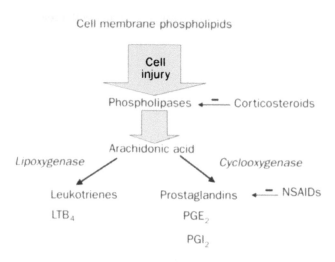

Figure 5.2 *Injury to tissue leads to the release of phospholipases, which in turn produce arachidonic acid. This pathway can be interrupted by the use of corticosteroids. The arachidonic acid may then lead to the production of leukotrienes such as LTB_4 by the lipoxygenase pathway or the production of endoperoxides such as prostaglandins (PGE_2 and PGI_2) and thromboxane A_2 by the cyclooxygenase pathway. This prostaglandin activity can be prevented by the use of non-steroidal anti-inflammatory drugs (NSAIDs).*

Table 5.2 Inflammatory mediators and their functions

Mediator	Effect
TNF-α	Releases IL-1, IL-6, IL-8, leukotrienes, thromboxane A_2, PGs; increases phagocytic activity of polymorphonuclear leukocytes
IL-1	Releases TNF-α, IL-6, IL-8, leukotrienes, PGs, thromboxane A_2; activates T cells and increases tissue cell sensitivity to TNF-α
IL-2	Releases TNF-α and leads to the proliferation of activated T cells
IL-6	Augments the proliferation and activation of T cells
IL-8	Chemotactic for neutrophils and lymphocytes
PAF	Stimulates release of TNF-α, leukotrienes, thromboxane A_2; alters microvascular permeability
LTB_4	Increases neutrophil chemotaxis and microvascular permeability
Thromboxane A_2	Increases PGI_2 production and platelet aggregation
PGE_2	Inhibits IL-1 release; induces vasodilatation; increases cAMP; with PGI_2, increases effects of 5-HT and BK
PGI2	Inhibits platelet aggregation and thrombus formation
BK	Promotes release of PGI_2

TNF-α, tumour necrosis factor α; IL, interleukin; PAF, platelet-activating factor; LTB_4, leukotriene B_4; PG, prostaglandin; BK, bradytrinin.

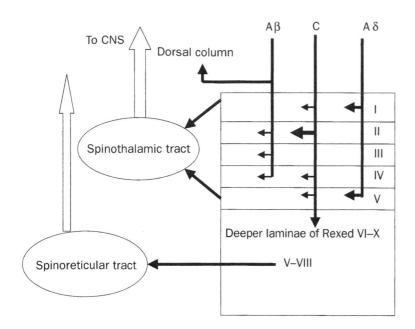

Figure 5.3 *Schematic diagram illustrating the destination of Aβ, Aδ, and C fibres within the lamina of Rexed, in the dorsal horn of the spinal cord. Heavier arrows indicate that the majority of fibres terminate at these points. There are many interneurones at various lamina, communicating between the laminae, which are normally involved in modulating sensory traffic but, following nerve injury, can be involved in perpetuating neuropathic pain. The neurones within the laminae project their signals to one of several tracts on the contralateral side of the spinal cord, before nociceptive information is conveyed to higher centres within the central nervous system (CNS).*

mechanoreceptors. From this point onwards, the sensory and nociceptive information tends to follow certain 'classical' pathways to higher centres in the CNS (Figure 5.3).

The axonal transport of this information is markedly influenced by many interconnecting neurones – within lamina I there are marginal cells, and within lamina II stalked and islet cells, together with projection neurones at lamina V. Wide-dynamic-range neurones (WDR) are found in laminae I, V, and VI. They can be activated by innocuous as well as noxious stimuli (light touch, pressure, pinch, or squeeze), so these sensations can be conveyed by Aβ, Aδ, or C fibres. Although Aβ fibres are associated with touch, they can influence nociception (see the discussion of the gate theory of pain later). These low-threshold fibres terminate at laminae II, III, and IV. Twenty-five percent of lamina II neurones are inhibitory, using the γ-amino-butyric acid (GABA) receptors A and B (GABA$_A$ and GABA$_B$). Lamina III information is perceived as non-noxious, typically from mechano-receptors and Pacini's corpuscles. Neurones in lamina IV extend to laminae I and II, receiving non-noxious afferent information. Lamina V contains largely WDR cells responding to non-

noxious stimuli and noxious high-threshold stimuli, which are conveyed to the contralateral spinothalamic tract.

All sensory information has the capacity to elicit reflex motor activity at the same spinal segmental level via interconnecting neurones, exiting the cord at the anterior root. This reflex action is an unconscious activity that, although protective in most instances, is not intended to reach consciousness. There are several main spinal tracts involved in nociception. Information from laminae I and V ascends by the spinothalamic tract, which is on the contralateral side of the cord to the afferent fibres conducting the nociceptive information. This tract projects to the ventrobasal thalamus and hence on to the somatosensory cortex. A further projection runs to the periaqueductal grey with descending information via dorsolateral funiculas to modulate incoming nociceptive traffic at the dorsal horn. The spinoreticular tract conveys nociceptive information from laminae V, VI, VII, and VIII. This tract passes through the reticular formation, from whence it projects to the hypothalamus, periaqueductal grey, and prefrontal cortex (Figure 5.4).

HIGHER CNS PATHWAYS

The spinal cord relays nociceptive information to the thalamic areas such as the ventrobasal complex and the reticular formation via two main systems: the paleospinothalamic tract, which is located medially in the cord and contains multiple synapses along its route, and the neospinothalamic tract, which is located laterally in the cord, without multiple relays along the way. The latter system is therefore capable of transmitting information more rapidly to higher levels in the CNS than the former system. Sensory information from Aβ fibres is also conveyed to the thalamus via the dorsal columns and their nuclei. It is only when nociceptive information reaches areas at or above the reticular formation that there is a conscious awareness of potential or actual tissue damage occurring.

There is a huge exchange of information between the reticular formation, hypothalamus, and thalamic nuclei. Further projections take place to the prefrontal cortex and the limbic system, which may augment the intensity or unpleasantness of the nociception, depending on affect and past experience. Despite these multiple communications, localisation of the site of nociception is not possible until the information reaches the somatosensory cortex. Other projections to the periaqueductal grey, amygdala, locus coeruleus, rostral medulla, and pons are involved in a feedback system, reducing the intensity of the sensation (Figure 5.4). These latter areas when stimulated induce analgesia by endorphin release, as well as through serotoninergic and noradrenergic pathways. Descending inhibitory control comes from the periaqueductal grey via the dorsolateral funiculus in the cord to the lamina I marginal zone. Many of these spinal pathways have been identified by horseradish peroxidase tracers, whereas mediators of analgesia or nociception are often identified by microinjection of various agonists. The use of functional magnetic resonance imaging (fMRI) has been another useful tool. It has indicated that parts of the motor cortex and the cerebellum are activated during nociception, despite the fact that no movement is involved at the time of the scan. These findings have been replicated, but their meaning remains unknown.

NEUROMODULATION AND THE GATE-CONTROL THEORY OF PAIN

Although pain pathways have been identified, there is a need to explain why a fixed stimulus does not result in a consistent response. From research carried out over the past 40 years, it is clear that there is a complex interplay between many structures within the CNS. In 1965, Melzack and Wall proposed that the fast-conducting Aβ fibres, normally involved in touch sensation, had the capacity to modulate afferent nociceptive information by a series of interneurones (Figure 5.5). This was described as a 'gate-control' system. Aβ-fibre activity could close the gate to C-fibre activity. Supraspinal influences, as mentioned above, were also able to modulate the nociceptive information (Figure 5.6). For instance, distraction could diminish the perception of pain, whereas anxiety or memory of an unpleasant situation during nociception could intensify it. Although the original theory was not completely correct, it went a long way towards explaining basic neuromodulation.

CHEMISTRY WITHIN THE SPINAL CORD

The transmission of nociceptive information, although dependent on electrical activity within the axon, requires the release of various neurotransmitters for interneuronal communication. A large variety of substances are used as neurotransmitters, ranging from protons (H^+) to larger molecules, such as amino acids and peptides.

Cations

Cations are positively charged ions such as H^+, Na^+, K^+, and Ca^{2+}. Some of these are released at the site of tissue damage peripherally (H^+ and K^+) and are responsible for direct excitation of the neurone. The exogenous administration of these substances results in a sharp, stinging, but transient sensation. Axonal conduction is by means of Na^+ channels, which can be inactivated by local anaesthetics. Some sensory neurones exhibit a long-lasting hyperpolarization, which is due to a cyclic guanosine monophosphate (cGMP)-dependent potassium conduction system.

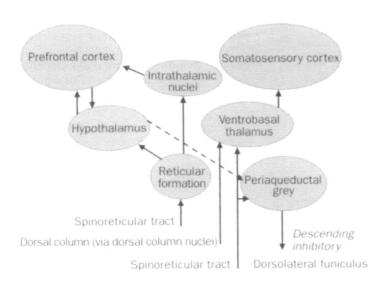

Figure 5.4 *Schematic diagram illustrating the main centres within the brain to which nociceptive traffic is conveyed, together with the intercommunications between these centres.*

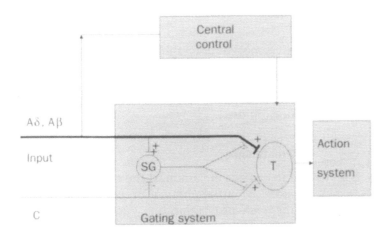

Figure 5.5 *The basis of the gate theory of pain in its simplest form, described by Melzack and Wall in 1965. Large myelinated fibres Aδ and Aβ signal to the substantia gelatinosa (SG) in lamina II to produce inhibitory messages as all nociceptive fibres communicate with the trigger cell (T), before this reaches higher centres and the motor responses (action system). Messages reaching higher centres in the central nervous system (central control) may result in descending inhibitory signals, further dampening the nociceptive information. (Reprinted with permission from Melzack R, Wall P. Science 1965; **150**: 971 (Figure 4).)*

Intracellular Ca^{2+} concentrations are controlled by voltage-dependent T, N, and L calcium channels. The N and L channels can be blocked by a number of substances, including opioids, GABA, and neuropeptide Y. The N calcium channel is particularly important as it is involved in both peripheral and central neuromodulation.

Nitric oxide

Nitric oxide (NO) also plays an important role in peripheral and central neuromodulation. Peripherally, it induces a delayed burning pain. Cofactors such as Ca^{2+} activate nitric oxide synthase (NOS) to form NO from L-arginine, which is found mostly in small and medium-sized neurones. NO alters intracellular processes mainly by the activation of guanylate cyclase. This is associated with an increase in the production of cGMP and is important in intracellular signalling. In addition, NO alters the responsiveness of sensory neurones to inflammatory substances such as bradykinin (BK), this appearing to be dependent on cGMP in the regulation of BK receptor–effector coupling mechanisms. Within

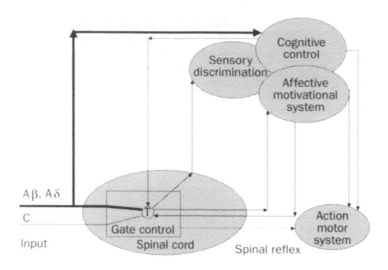

Figure 5.6 *Interrelationship between modulating systems in the spinal cord, cognitive control, and the affective motivational system. These cognitive and affective systems can have profound inhibitory effects on the perception of pain, or may indeed augment the signal depending on the meaning of pain at the time of nociception and past experiences.*

the spinal cord, constituitive NOS may also be stimulated by N-methyl-D-aspartate (NMDA)-induced activity, generating sufficient NO to produce cytotoxicity.

Bradykinin

When tissue damage occurs, kininogens are converted to kallikreins to BK and kallidin, both of which are rapidly degraded by kininases to generate the inactive metabolites: des-Arg-bradykinin or des-Arg-kallidin respectively. At least two classes of kinin receptor have been identified: B_1 and B_2.

The pro-inflammatory effects generated by BK are:

- plasma extravasation by Ca^{2+}-dependent activation of contractile proteins on venular endothelial cells;
- release of prostaglandins and cytokinins from various cells;
- stimulation of postganglionic sympathetic neurones to release prostanoids, which sensitise afferent neurones and alter blood vessel diameter, which is important in plasma extravasation;
- degranulation of mast cells, releasing inflammatory mediators such as histamine.

- chemotaxis of lymphocytes to the site of injury.

BK is a most potent endogenous algogenic substance, also inducing direct stimulation of nociceptors.

Prostanoids

Prostanoids are amongst the most potent mediators of inflammatory hyperalgesia – they include prostaglandins, leukotrienes, and hydroxy acids. They act at a number of receptors, coupling with second messengers. Prostaglandins do not normally induce pain when injected intradermally – rather they sensitise sensory neurones by reducing their activation threshold and enhancing their response to other stimuli. Prostaglandins are widely distributed throughout the body and are normally generated as the consistitutive forms of cyclooxygenase (COX-1) and serve a number of physiological functions. During inflammation, prostaglandin formation is enhanced by the induction of another form of the enzyme, COX-2. NSAIDs block the actions of COX enzymes, but those drugs that selectively block COX-2 produce analgesia without the gastric or haematological side-effects widely associated with this class of substance.

Adenosine triphosphate

Adenosine triphosphate (ATP) activates sensory neurones, increasing their permeability to ions, and when this substance is injected intradermally it produces short transient pain. The degradation product of ATP, adenosine, also provokes pain and hyperalgesia when administered intradermally. This activity is due to activation of adenosine A_2 receptors, which are coupled with adenosine cyclase. The production of cyclic adenosine monophosphate (cAMP) and the reduction of K^+ permeability accounts for the hyperexcitability in afferent fibres. However, adenosine may also activate A_1 receptors, which negatively couple to cAMP activation, reducing afferent excitability. This causes a block in Ca^{2+} conductance or increased K^+ permeability, resulting in antinociception.

Histamine

When mast cells degranulate, histamine and other inflammatory mediators are released. These produce itching at low concentrations and pain at higher concentrations. Sensory neurones express histamine H_1 receptors, the activation of which increases membrane Ca^{2+} permeability. This in turn releases sensory neuropeptides as well as prostaglandins, leading to hyperalgesia and other pro-inflammatory effects.

Serotonin

Like ATP, serotonin (5-hydroxytryptamine, 5-HT) can cause direct excitation of sensory neurones by increasing Na^+ permeability. This is due to activation of the $5\text{-}HT_3$ receptor. A similar effect may occur when serotonin is released from platelets and mast cells during injury or inflammation, since the $5\text{-}HT_3$ receptor binding site is part of a cation-selective channel. The effect may be produced through the Na^+ channel. It is known that serotonin activates sensory neurones by G-protein-coupled $5\text{-}HT_1$ and $5\text{-}HT_2$ receptors. This induces a decrease in K^+ permeability and a membrane polarisation that may sensitise nociceptors and lower their threshold to heat and pressure stimuli, and can even induce repetitive neurone firing.

Nerve growth factor

Nerve growth factor (NGF) is one of a number of substances that play a specific role in the development, maintenance, and regeneration of peripheral nerve fibres. It is a protein normally produced by cells in target organs such as skin and blood vessels. When secreted, it is taken up by sympathetic and small sensory fibres to be transported retrogradely to the cell body. Failure of NGF production results in nerve degeneration and, if nerve destruction occurs, results in abnormal sensation. This is partly due to a reduced expression of neuropeptides such as SP and calcitonin gene-related peptide (CGRP). Such a failure also results in autonomic failure and adrenergic sympathetic dysfunction. An excessive production of NGF, on the other hand, produces hyperalgesia such as that found in inflammation. A number of different lesions may result in an inadequate supply of NGF to sensory neurones, including the removal of target organs normally secreting the factor, or damage to the nerve, which can prevent axonal transport of NGF. Damage to a peripheral nerve results in increased synthesis of NGF due to upregulation. This has been attributed to factors which are released by invading macrophages, including interleukin-1 (IL-1). If regeneration of a nerve occurs, the target tissue is able to supply sufficient NGF to restore an adequate supply of SP so that the sensory fibre may function normally. Damaged nerves usually send out sprouts, which have increased susceptibility to NGF, resulting in hyperalgesia. It has been postulated that failure of the spinal cord to adapt to the lack of incoming NGF results in some chronic pain states such as that seen in post-herpetic neuralgia. The changes in NGF seen in the early stages of nerve injury appear to play an essential role in the adaptive response of the nerve, but can potentially lead to chronic pain.

Substance P

SP is a undecapeptide and is found in the dorsal horn of the spinal cord but originates from primary afferent fibres. Peripheral noxious stimuli result in the release of SP, which has a peripheral effect on the polymodal nociceptor, both increasing its sensitivity to further noxious stimuli and triggering an inflammatory response. During inflammation, there is a marked increase in neuropeptide content within the primary afferent. Substances like galanin and somatostatin reduce neurogenic inflammation by lowering primary afferent excitability. Other substances such as noradrenaline increase the excitability of primary afferents; this is especially evident following nerve injury.

NEUROMODULATION

When the primary afferent has been stimulated, a complex series of interactions take place within the dorsal horn of the spinal cord. Although the nociceptive information could potentially be transmitted through to the spinothalamic tract without modification, interneurones produce substances that can augment or inhibit the nociceptor traffic. Within the dorsal horn, glutamate and aspartate from interneurones excite second-order neurones and augment nociception. Somatostatin, CGRP, vasoactive intestinal polypeptide (VIP), and neurotensin may also augment nociceptor transmission. At the primary synapses glutamate excitation is mediated by non-NMDA receptors, such as the AMPA (α-amino-3-hydroxy-5-methyl-4-isoxazole propionate) receptor. However, excitation of second-order neurones by glutamate is via the NMDA receptor.

Inhibition of nociception occurs through interneurones releasing enkephalin, mainly at laminae I, II, and V. These endogenous opioids acts at receptors located presynaptically at the terminals of primary afferents and at the postsynaptic neurone. GABA is another potent inhibitor of nociception and is found in lamina II. It is involved in presynaptic inhibition. Descending inhibitory fibres from the CNS use noradrenaline and serotonin to inhibit or reduce nociceptive traffic.

'WIND-UP' AND CENTRAL SENSITIZATION

In animal experiments, it has been illustrated that the firing of C fibres at a critical high frequency (typically 0.5 Hz) causes a normal response for a few seconds followed by an exponential build-up in the electrophysiological activity of dorsal horn neurones. This activity is called 'wind-up' and leads to an expansion of the receptive fields of that spinal cord segment, since a wide variety of neurones are affected. The phenomenon occurs only under certain conditions in a laboratory situation and helps to explain why spinal cord sensitisation occurs.

Wind-up is not a clinical phenomenon but rather a situation that occurs in experimental circumstances. Spinal cord or central sensitisation is the clinical manifestation of an ongoing pain situation mediated by excitatory amino acids. These changes are known to be mediated by the NMDA receptor. Excitatory amino acids such as glycine and aspartate can trigger the NMDA receptor, which is normally blocked by Mg^{2+} to prevent a Ca^{2+} influx (Figure 5.7). When the Mg^{2+} plug is displaced, Ca^{2+} can rapidly enter the neurone, triggering an increased concentration of protein kinase C (PKC). This in turn leads to further sensitisation of the postsynaptic cell (Figure 5.8). If the stimulation is particularly intense, the resulting activity leads to an increase in intracellular NO, alteration in gene transcription, and ultimately changes in the neurotransmitters produced. These changes are expressed by immediate early genes including the c-*fos* and c-*jun* proto-oncogenes. These bind to some DNA sequences and regulate the transcription of target genes (Figure 5.9). If the intracellular concentrations of Ca^{2+} become particularly high, cell death can ensue. This excitation occurs rapidly when mediated via the AMPA receptor and more slowly via the NMDA receptor. The timescales of some of these mediators are generalised in Table 5.3.

NEUROPATHIC PAIN

When tissue insult occurs, nociception occurs for seconds to days, depending on the degree of damage and how rapidly the inflammatory mediators are removed. Under some circumstances, pain may persist for months or years even when the injured tissues have healed. This perpetuation of pain is thought to be due to CNS

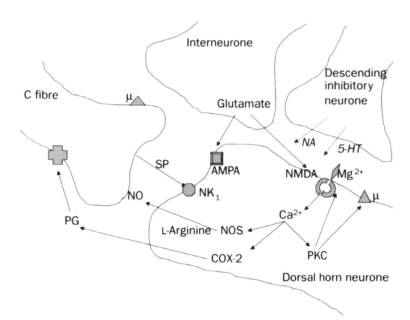

Figure 5.7 *Modulating systems within the dorsal horn as the terminal primary afferent is signalling second-order neurones (dorsal horn neurone). The release of neurotransmitters from the C fibre stimulates the NK_1 receptor. In addition, the release of the excitatory amino acid glutamate stimulates the α-amino-3-hydroxy-5-methyl-4-isoxazole propionate (AMPA) and N-methyl-D-aspartate (NMDA) receptors, with a resulting influx of Ca^{2+} into the dorsal horn neurone. This in turn induces the release of cyclooxygenase-2 (COX-2), nitric oxide (NO), and protein kinase C (PKC). This sensitises the C fibre via the prostaglandin receptor (PG). (NA, noradrenaline; 5-HT, serotonin; NOS, NO synthase; SP, substance P.)*

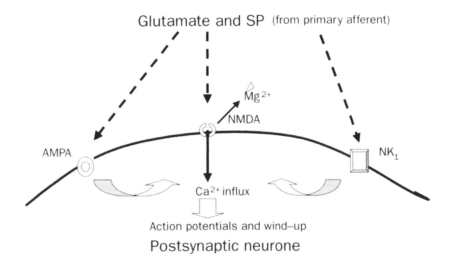

Figure 5.8 *The mechanism of wind-up: glutamate activation of the AMPA receptor, compared with the moderate onset time at the NMDA receptor. If the NK_1 receptor is activated by substance P (SP) as well as glutamate activating the NMDA receptor, Mg^{2+} blocking this receptor is displaced, allowing an influx of Ca^{2+}. Depending on the extent of Ca^{2+} influx, this can result in large action potentials or an ongoing state of excitation. (Based on Goodchild CS. Pain Rev 1997; 4: 33–58. Reprinted with permission by Arnold Publishers.)*

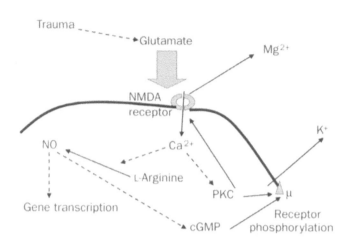

Figure 5.9 *Opioid intolerance frequently occurs after nerve damage due to central sensitisation, mediated by the NMDA receptor. Altered cell chemistry results in phosphorylation of the proteins at the μ receptor, reducing their sensitivity to both exogenous opioids such as morphine in addition to the endogenous opioids (enkephalin). (Based on Goodchild CS.* Pain Rev *1997;* **4:** *33–58. Reprinted with permission by Arnold Publishers.)*

Table 5.3 Excitation timescales

Mediator	Onset time	Duration
AMPA	Milliseconds	Milliseconds
NMDA	Milliseconds	Years
SP, CGRP	Milliseconds	Hours
Ca^{2+}, NO, PKC, PG	Milliseconds	Days
c-fos, c-jun	Minutes	Years
CCK, growth factors	Hours	Years

AMPA, α-amino-3-hydroxy-5-methyl-4-isoxazole propionate; NMDA, *N*-methyl-D-aspartate; SP, substance P; CGRP, calcitonin gene-related peptide; NO, nitric oxide; PKC, protein kinase C; PG, prostaglandin; CCK, cholecystokinin.

changes or in some situations to sympathetic–sensory coupling: sympathetically maintained pain (Figure 5.10). Neuropathic pain is therefore a malfunction of the transmission system – typically a primary lesion or dysfunction of the nervous system. This can occur not only due to nerve trauma but also as a result of some diseases, such as diabetes mellitus, herpes zoster, CNS neoplasms, CNS infarct, and multiple sclerosis. Sometimes the pain may occur without an obvious initiating factor (e.g. trigeminal neuralgia) and may be initiated intermittently without obvious initialling factors. Since the transmission of normal sensory information, such as touch, is altered, its perception is often perceived as unpleasant.

Dysaesthesia is an unpleasant sensation, often felt as tingling or a shooting. Allodynia occurs after nerve injury and is a painful sensation in response to a non-noxious stimulus, mediated by Aδ fibres (e.g. touching an area of skin that has just been burned). When a normally noxious stimulus results in an exaggerated response, hyperalgesia is said to exist. Many of these perceptions will occur within minutes after injury due to the effect of inflammatory mediators such as BK and serotonin. Their effect should not persist unless there is a central mechanism,

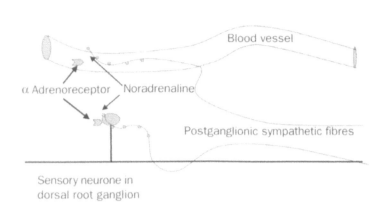

Figure 5.10 *Following peripheral nerve injury, coupling of sensory and sympathetic neurones occurs in the dorsal root ganglion as well as at the site of nerve injury. This, together with a possible upregulation of α adrenoreceptors, increases neurone responsiveness to endogenous noradrenaline. Vasoconstriction also occurs, leading to tropic tissue changes and reduced perfusion of the nerve, exacerbating the pain situation.*
(Based on Michaelis M. Proceedings of the 9th World Congress on Pain. Seattle: IASP Press, 2000: 645–56. Reprinted with permission.)

such as the situations where intensive stimulation may result in alteration in CNS chemistry due, in the long term, to gene expression.

When a peripheral nerve is damaged, usually by trauma, changes as shown in Figure 5.9 occur, with an influx of Ca^{2+} triggering many long-term changes in the primary afferent and second-order neurones. These in turn may result in opioid insensitivity. Approximately 70% of the μ receptors in the spinal cord are thought to be at presynaptic sites of the terminal afferents, and there is a downregulation of these and the number of sites. At the postsynaptic neurone, sensitisation of the cell may be such that phosphorylation of the μ receptor takes place, rendering it relatively ineffective to exogenous as well as endogenous opioids, such as endorphin. Other inhibitory mechanisms may also become less effective, such as noradrenaline, serotonin, and the GABA receptors. In these situations, the use of drugs active within the CNS has been successfully employed, such as:

- tricyclic antidepressants – these boost the reuptake of neurotransmitters used by the inhibitory pathways;
- sodium channel blockers (e.g. carbamazepine), which are active on the neurone, stabilizing it;
- calcium channel blockers (e.g. gabapentin), which are active on the neurone, stabilizing it;
- baclofen, which is active at the GABA receptor;
- cannabinoids, which are active at K^+, Na^+, Ca^{2+}, serotonin, and adenylate cyclase sites.

Cannabinoids appear to have antihyperalgesic effects at peripheral and central terminals of primary afferent neurones (CB_1 and CB_2 receptor sites). Receptor sites for these substances at the periaqueductal grey and the rostral ventromedial medulla mediate antinociception.

When nerve injury occurs, some primary afferents express functional α_2 adrenoreceptors (Figure 5.10). These receptors may be present on the nerve, but in a non-functional state, until triggered. SP is known to express α_2 adrenoreceptors in the intact DRG, but these normally have an inhibitory role. Neuropeptide Y, which itself is a sympathetic transmitter, enhances the excitability of the DRG neurones after injury through Y_2 receptors, by the attenuation of Ca^{2+}-dependent K^+ conductance in the cell. Sympathetic–sensory coupling can occur at the site of injury, where sprouting of nerve fibres occurs at the site of a neuroma. These sprouts are atypical, being unusually responsive to endogenous noradrenaline and local mechanical stimulation. In addition, there is evidence of direct sympathetic–sensory coupling at the site of injury, with further sympathetic–sensory coupling occurring at the dorsal root ganglion. The increase in catecholamines may not only directly stimulate the primary afferent but also increase its sensitivity by hypoperfusion of the nerve and surrounding tissues. Sympathetic blockade can therefore be a valuable therapeutic option in this situation (Figure 5.11).

VISCERAL PAIN

The viscera, such as the thoracic and abdominal contents, have a relatively low number of afferents compared with the skin. Innervation is by C fibres, which form a nerve plexus. From here, the nociceptive information combines with somatic afferents: the somato-visceral convergence. This mixing of visceral and somatic afferents occurs mainly at the low thoracic region, accounting for over 60% of all neurones (splanchnic nerves), the remainder being in the lower cervical area. The preganglionic sympathetic fibres utilise acetylecholine for neurotransmission whereas the postganglionic neurotransmission is with noradrenaline.

The somatic representation of visceral nociception tends to be at the following sites:

- heart: T1 – T6 and C2 – C4;
- stomach: T6 – T9;
- pancreas: T6 – T10;
- kidney: T10 – L1;
- rectum: S2 – S4.

Structures between the diaphragm and the pelvis send nociceptive information by the sympathetic nervous system. Some intrathoracic structures, including the heart, also convey nociceptive information by this means. Pain originating in the oesophagus, trachea, and pharynx is conveyed centrally by the parasympathetic nervous system. Deep pelvic structures such as the rectum, testis, cervix, upper vagina, and trigone of the bladder are also innervated by parasympathetic nerves.

The visceral C fibres are high-threshold afferents, responding to the distension of hollow organs or prolonged stimulation of the viscera, due to tissue hypoxia or inflammation. Many of these afferents are 'silent' nociceptors, only becoming active during episodes of inflammation or ischaemia, when kinins and other inflammatory mediators are released from damaged cells. This results in switching silent nociceptors to active ones, responding to mechanical stimulation. Viscerosomatic neurones in the spinal cord are nociceptive-specific, some being low-threshold, wide-dynamic-range cells. Most are located in laminae I and V, with a much smaller number in laminae II, III, and IV. The nociceptive information travels by the spinothalamic and spinoreticular tracts, inducing thalamic and hypothalamic stimulation. It also has a major impact on brainstem areas associated with the autoregulation of breathing and blood pressure. The vagus nerve is important in the central transmission of parasympathetic information; 80% of the fibres are afferent and although most of this information does not reach consciousness, it is capable of carrying nociceptive information. This is via the nucleus of the solitary tract (glutamatergic neurones) and the parabrachial nucleus (NMDA receptors) to the ventral basal thalamus, hypothalamus, and brainstem. The incoming signals are modulated by GABA and α_2 receptors, together with noradrenergic neurones.

The primary somatosensory cortex receives very little visceral input, but the ventrolateral orbital cortex does – an area associated with aversive and emotional aspects of pain. Therefore, in addition to visceral pain being associated with somatic structures, it tends to:

- be poorly localized;
- generate regional or whole-body motor responses;
- cause strong autonomic responses;
- produce strong affective responses;
- cause nausea.

This type of pain responds best to opioid analgesics and sympathetic blockade of the appropriate nerve plexus if the pain is chronic. It responds poorly if at all to most other forms of analgesia, since there is a notable upregulation of the immediate early gene c-*fos*, and this responds well to μ agonists and NMDA receptor antagonists.

SUMMARY

Although precise sensory and nociceptive pathways have been identified, these cannot be accepted as the only 'pain pathways'. Interruption of these often only stops or min-

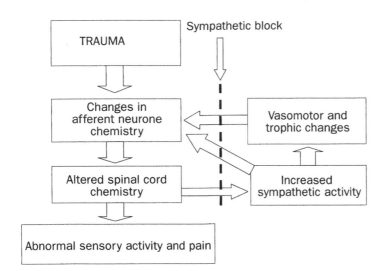

Figure 5.11 *The potential mechanism by which sympathetic blockade can reduce sympathetically maintained pain, such as that seen in complex regional pain syndromes.*

imises pain for a matter of months. There is a complex communication between neurones at many levels within the CNS, from the point of the first synapses through to higher centres in the brain. Processing of this information is constantly changing (plasticity of the CNS), due to mood, distraction, etc. Nociceptive pain generally resolves in hours to weeks, as healing of tissues occurs and peripheral inflammatory mediators diminish with time. Neuropathic pain is much more difficult to manage due to complex systems coming into play, with changes in gene transcription and the resulting changes in neurone behaviour. This latter problem remains a challenge to medical practice.

FURTHER READING

Melzack R, Wall PD. Pain mechanisms: a new theory. *Science* 1965; **150**: 971–9.

Koltzenburg M. Neural mechanisms of cutaneous nociceptive pain. *Clin J Pain* 2000; **16**: S131–8.

Mannion RJ, Woolf CJ. Pain mechanisms and management: a central perspective. *Clin J Pain* 2000; **16**: S144–56.

Wall P. *Pain. The Science of Suffering*. London: Weidenfeld & Nicolson, 2000.

Yaksh TL. Spinal systems and pain processing: development of novel analgesic drugs with mechanistically defined models. *Trends Pharmacol Sci* 1999; **20**: 329–37.

Berger A. Phantoms in the brain. *BMJ* 1999; **319**: 587–8.

Cervero F. Mechanisms of visceral pain: past and present. In: *Visceral Pain* (Gerhart GH, ed). Seattle: IASP Press, 1995: 25–40.

Janig W, Habler H-J. Visceral–autonomic integration. In: *Visceral Pain* (Gerhart GH, ed). Seattle: IASP Press, 1995: 311–48.

Goodchild CS. Nonopioid spinal analgesics: animal experimentation and implications for clinical developments. *Pain Rev* 1997; **4**: 33–58.

Michaelis M. Coupling of sympathetic and somatosensory neurons following nerve injury: mechanisms and potential significance for the generation of pain. In: *Proceedings of the 9th World Congress on Pain* (Devor M, Rowbotham MC, Wiesenfeld-Hallin Z, eds). Seattle: IASP Press, 2000: 645–56.

6

Red blood cells, haemostasis, and white blood cells

Nollag O'Rourke, George Shorten

RED BLOOD CELLS

General properties

The red blood cell (RBC) is unique among eukaryotic cells in that its principal physical structure is its membrane, which encloses a concentrated haemoglobin solution. Unlike other cells, the RBC has no cytoplasmic structures or organelles, and does not have a nucleus.

The average RBC count is 4.5–$6.5 \times 10^{12}/l$ in men and 3.8–$5.8 \times 10^{12}/l$ in women, each cell containing 27–32 pg of haemoglobin (Table 6.1). Mature erythrocytes are biconcave discs 7–8 µm in diameter, 2.5 µm thick at the rim, and 1 µm at the centre. The geometry of the RBC, the viscosity of its intracellular milieu, and the material properties of its membrane allow it to pass through 3 µm capillaries and 2–3 µm slits in the reticuloendothelial sinusoids. The large surface area-to-volume ratio also facilitates diffusion of respiratory gases across its membrane.

The RBC membrane is composed of a lipid bilayer to which two main groups of proteins (peripheral and integral) are attached. The peripheral proteins form a filamentous network, anchored to the cytoplasmic surface of the bilayer, constituting the membrane cytoskeleton. This is essential for maintaining shape and regulating the membrane properties of deformability and mechanical stability. These proteins include spectrin, actin, protein 4.1, pallidan, anchorin, adductin, tropomyosin and tropomodulin. Defects of this protein cytoskeleton are responsible for inherited abnormalities of erythrocyte shape, for example hereditary spherocytosis and elliptocytosis. Acquired defects of the RBC membrane also cause anaemia such as paroxysmal nocturnal haemoglobinuria.

The integral proteins span the membrane. Band 3 (anion exchanger), aquaporin 1 (water channel), and glycophorins are the most abundant proteins of this class. They provide binding sites for several glycolytic enzymes and provide transport facilities for bicarbonate (HCO_3^-) and water (e.g. aquaporin 1). Other integral proteins include Na^+/K^+-ATPase and a Ca^{2+}/Mg^{2+}-ATPase, which mediate active ion transport across the cell membrane.

RBC metabolism

As the RBC has no cytochrome system, it is incapable of complete oxidative phosphorylation or of sustaining the Krebs cycle. Therefore, ATP is produced by glycolysis. Unlike other cells, glucose entry to the RBC is not dependent on binding of insulin to specific insulin receptors. Glycolysis also provides the RBC with a supply of reduced nicotinamide adenine dinucleotide (NADH). NADH is a coenzyme for a reductase enzyme that maintains the iron of haemoglobin in the ferrous state (Fe^{2+}). If the iron is oxidised to the ferric state (Fe^{3+}), the methaemoglobin (MetHb) so formed cannot combine reversibly with oxygen.

Approximately 5–10% of the glucose metabolised

Table 6.1. Red blood cell (RBC) indices

RBC index		Men	Women
RBC count		$4.5–6.5 \times 10^{12}/l$	$3.8–5.8 \times 10^{12}/l$
Haemoglobin concentration (Hb)		13–18 g/dl	11.5–16.5 g/dl
Haematocrit (packed cell volume) (Hct)		0.40–0.54	0.37–0.47
Mean cell volume	$\dfrac{Hct \times 10}{RBC(10^{12}/l)}$	76–96 fl	76–96 fl
Mean cell haemoglobin	$\dfrac{Hb \times 10}{RBC(10^{12}/l)}$	27–32 pg	27–32 pg
Mean cell haemoglobin concentration	$\dfrac{Hb \times 100}{Hct}$	30–35 g/dl	30–35 g/dl
Reticulocyte count		$25–85 \times 10^9/l$	$25–85 \times 10^9/l$
Reticulocyte count (%)		0.2–2.0	0.2–2.0

by the red cell is diverted via the hexose mono-phosphate shunt (pentose phosphate pathway) during which NADP is reduced to NADPH. Methaemogloblin may also be reduced by the coenzyme NADPH. The reducing power of NADPH is made available to the cell through its linkage with glutathione. The reducing agent also provides protection against the oxidation of sulfhydryl groups of enzymes, globin, and constituents of the membrane.

A side-reaction of the glycolytic pathway leads to the synthesis of 2,3-diphosphoglycerate (2,3-DPG). This binds with haemoglobin to decrease its affinity for oxygen, thus promoting release of oxygen to the tissues. Conditions causing hypoxia, such as high altitude or severe anaemia, promote production of 2,3-DPG.

Deficiencies in RBC enzymes can lead to increased destruction of the RBC and anaemia – for example glucose-6-phosphate dehydrogenase (G6PD) deficiency. This enzyme catalyses the first step in the oxidation of glucose via the hexose monophosphate shunt. The gene for G6PD resides on the X chromosome and therefore the condition is inherited as a sex-linked characteristic. When providing anaesthetic care for these patients, it important to avoid oxidant stress such as those imposed by high-dose aspirin, phenacetin, or sulfonamide administra-tion. Fortunately, few of these 'triggering' agents are currently used in anaesthetic practice.

RBC production

Erythropoiesis entails mitosis and maturation of the primitive stem cell in the bone marrow with release of reticulocytes into the bloodstream. The proerythroblast is the earliest recognizable RBC precursor. It is formed from stem cells in the bone marrow under the influence of ery-thropoietin (EPO). The cells divide and mature to form the reticulocyte. This process involves a decrease in cell size, nuclear condensation and extrusion, and haemoglobin accumulation. In acute anaemia, the duration of this process is shortened. Reticulocytes mature for 1–2 days in the bloodstream, losing their remaining ribo-somes to become mature RBC.

EPO (MW 33 000 Da), which has a half-life of 5 hours, is secreted from the kidney in response to tissue hypoxia. About 10–15% is produced in the liver. Other known haematopoetic factors include interleukin-3 (IL-3), granulocyte–macrophage colony-stimulating factor (GM-CSF), steel factor (also known as stem cell factor (SCF) and c-Kit ligand), and hormones such as insulin, thyroxine, corticosteroids, and growth hormone.

HAEMOGLOBIN

General properties

Haemoglobin (MW 64 450Da), the oxygen-carrying pigment of the RBC, enables the transport of 20 ml oxygen per 100 ml blood (100 times more than could be transported in solution alone). It consists of four subunits, each containing a haem moiety conjugated to a polypeptide. Haem consists of a protoporphyrin ring with a central atom of ferrous iron (Fe^{2+}), which can combine reversibly with one molecule of oxygen. Each haemoglobin molecule can therefore bind as many as four oxygen molecules in separate chemical reactions. The change in molecular conformation induced by the binding of the first three oxygen molecules greatly accelerates binding of the fourth (hysteresis). This complex interaction between the haemoglobin subunits accounts for the characteristic sigmoid shape of the haemoglobin–oxygen dissociation curve.

There are four types of globin chains (α, β, γ, and δ) which differ in their constituent amino acids. HbA, containing two α and two β chains, comprises 96–98% of adult haemoglobin. Adults also have 2–3% HbA_2 (two α and two δ chains) and 1% fetal haemoglobin HbF (2α and 2γ). Human fetal blood contains HbF, which is normally replaced by adult haemoglobin 3–6 months after birth. Fetal Hb has a greater affinity for oxygen than adult haemoglobin, and this is reflected in a leftward shift of the oxygen dissociation curve. In the fetal circulation, the oxygen content of blood at a given P_{aO_2} is greater than that in the adult. The increased affinity of HbF for oxygen facilitates transfer of oxygen from the maternal circulation to the fetal circulation. The downloading of oxygen to fetal tissues is inhibited by HbF, but compensatory mechanisms prevail, for example high haemoglobin concentration (17 g/dl), increased RBC count, large oxygen gradient, and shift of oxygen dissociation curve to the right (increased CO_2, increased 2,3-DPG).

Synthesis and catabolism of haemoglobin

In the bone marrow, haem and the globin moiety are synthesised separately before combining to form haemoglobin molecules in the primitive RBC. Amino acids are required for production of globin chains. The synthesis of haem requires iron, glycine, succinyl coenzyme A, and pyridoxine (vitamin B_6). Vitamin B_{12} and folic acid are required for DNA replication during RBC maturation. Deficiency in any of these can decrease haemoglobin production or erythropoiesis.

The lifespan of a RBC is approximately 120 days, after which it is removed from the circulation by the tissue macrophage system. Within the macrophage, the RBC is broken down, with the release and degradation of haemoglobin. The globin portion is cleaved off and its constituent amino acids returned to the general amino acid pool. Haem oxygenase converts haem to biliverdin, which in turn is converted to bilirubin and excreted in bile. The iron released is transported as transferrin either to the bone marrow, where it is incorporated into new haem groups, or to the liver. Carbon monoxide (CO) is a normal by-product of haem breakdown.

Variants of haemoglobin

Compared with O_2, CO has a 300 times greater affinity for haemoglobin, combining with it to form carboxyhaemoglobin (COHb). Carbon monoxide decreases the oxygen-carrying capacity of haemoglobin and causes a leftward shift in the oxygen dissociation curve, thereby decreasing oxygen delivery to the tissues. Pulse oximetry interprets COHb as 90% oxyHb and 10% deoxyHb. Therefore, at abnormally high levels of COHb, the oxygen saturation (S_{pO_2}) reading is an overestimate. Other clinically important factors that influence oxygen binding to haemoglobin include hydrogen ion concentration, 2,3-DPG concentration, temperature, and P_{aCO_2}.

Methaemogloblin results when the iron in haem is oxidized to its trivalent form (Fe^{3+}). Nitrates, nitrites, sulfonamides, and other drugs occasionally result in significant methaemoglobinaemia (defined as >1% of total Hb). Methaemoglobinaemia, like carbon monoxide poisoning, decreases the oxygen-carrying capacity of the blood and impairs release of oxygen to the tissues. Reduction of methaemoglobin is facilitated by such agents as methylene blue or ascorbic acid. In general, as the proportion of methaemoglobin increases, S_{pO_2} values approach 80–85%.

Sickle cell syndromes are inherited haemoglobinopathies resulting from a point mutation of the globin gene: substitution of valine for glutamic acid in the sixth position of the β chain. This transforms HbA to HbS, which on deoxygenation tends to undergo aggregation and polymerization leading to sickling of RBC. In heterozygotes (sickle cell trait), approximately 40% of the haemoglobin is HbS, which leads to sickling in conditions of severe hypoxia. Patients with sickle cell trait are at little risk during a properly conducted anaesthetic, although the use of a tourniquet is inadvisable. In contrast, sickle cell disease (homozygous $\alpha_2 S_2$ globin) is characterised by anaemia, chronic haemolysis, microvascular occlusions, and increased susceptibility to infections. Special precautions to prevent hypothermia, hypoxia, hypercarbia, dehydration, and acidosis must be taken perioperatively. Other sickle cell syndromes include the double heterozygous conditions, sickle C (HbSC) and sickle thalassaemia (HbSThal), in which the sickle cell gene is inherited in addition to another variant, such as HbC or β thalassaemia.

Single point mutations of haemoglobin can decrease the solubility of the molecule in the red cell (unstable haemoglobins). Two hundred and fifty known unstable mutations are described, including abnormalities of the α, β, and γ globin chains. The most common are Hb Köln (β98 Val→Met) and Hb Poole (γ130 Trp→Gly), which can cause haemolysis in the newborn.

Deficiency of haemoglobin – anaemia

Anaemia is an abnormal decrease in the proportionate volume of RBCs (as measured by the haematocrit), or an abnormal decrease in the haemoglobin concentration of the blood. The World Health Organisation defines anaemia as <13 g/dl in adult men, <12 g/dl in women, <11 g/dl in children aged 6 months to 6 years and <12 g/dl in children aged 6–14 years. Anaemia is classified according to RBC morphology or cause (Tables 6.2 and 6.3).

In the absence of compensation, anaemia results in a decrease in oxygen delivery to the tissues. Compensatory mechanisms include an increase in cardiac output, a decrease in blood viscosity, and an increase in 2,3-DPG. These mechanisms enhance the delivery of oxygen to the tissues – the third by shifting the oxyhaemoglobin dissociation curve to the right.

There is no universally accepted preoperative minimum haemoglobin concentration. Preoperative management depends on the cause, a patient's overall medical status (in particular, cardiac reserve), and the planned surgery.

BLOOD GROUPS

Human RBC membranes have at least 20 different antigenic systems, each under genetic control from a separate chromosomal locus. The ABO and Rhesus systems are important in the majority of blood transfusions. The chromosomal locus for the ABO system produces three alleles, which are inherited in a Mendelian dominant manner. Those with blood group A have A antigens on the surface of their RBC; those with group B have B antigens, those with group AB have both antigens, and those with group O have neither. These antigens are also found on other tissues, including salivary glands, saliva, pancreas, kidney, liver, lungs, testes, semen, and amniotic fluid.

On the surface of RBC, these antigens are glycosphingolipids, whereas on other cells, they are glycoproteins. The H antigen, which is present on the surface of all RBC in its modified form, is produced at a different chromosomal locus. Individuals with blood group A have a gene encoding a transferase that catalyses placement of a terminal N-acetylgalactosamine on the H antigen, whereas group B individuals have a gene encoding a transferase that places a terminal galactose. Individuals who are group AB have both transferases. Individuals who are type O have neither, in which case the H antigen persists in its unmodified form. Almost all individuals who do not express A or B antigens 'naturally' produce antibodies (IgM) against them in the first year of life (Table 6.4). Antibodies can also occur in response to sensitisation from a previous blood transfusion or pregnancy.

Table 6.2 Classification of anaemia according to red blood cell morphology

Type of anaemia[a]	Cause
Hypochromic, microcytic (decreased MCV, MCH, and MCHC)	Iron deficiency (deficiency of haem synthesis) Thalassaemias (deficiency of globin synthesis)
Normochromic, macrocytic (increased MCV) i.e. megaloblatic	Vitamin B_{12} deficiency Folate deficiency Alcohol
Polychromatic, macrocytic (increased MCV)	Haemolysis
Normocytic, normochromic	Chronic disease, renal failure, hypothyroidism, marrow aplasia or infiltration, acute haemorrhage
Leucoerythroblastic	Marrow infiltration

[a] MCV, mean cell volume, i.e. RBC size, which may be macrocytic (increased), microcytic (decreased), or normocytic (normal); MCH, mean corpuscular haemoglobin (average amount of haemoglobin in the cells); MCHC, mean corpuscular haemoglobin concentration (average concentration of haemoglobin in the cells).

Expression of the Rhesus antigen is regulated at three chromosomal loci with a total of six alleles, the most immunogenic being that which produces the D antigen. Approximately 80–85% of Caucasians express the D antigen. Individuals lacking this allele are Rh-negative and usually develop antibodies against the D antigen only after exposure to a previous (Rh-positive) transfusion or pregnancy (a Rh-negative mother delivering a Rh-positive baby). Fortunately, this latter disorder can easily be avoided by administration of anti-D immunoglobulin soon after delivery. This prevents sensitisation of maternal lymphocytes by any fetal RBC D antigen that may have been transferred across the placenta during parturition.

BLOOD TRANSFUSION

Transfusion reactions

The most dangerous transfusion reactions arise when naturally occurring antibodies (recipient serum) react with foreign antigen (donor cells), activating complement and resulting in intravascular haemolysis. The consequences of intravascular haemolysis range from mild jaundice (increased plasma bilirubin concentration) to renal tubular damage (from products of RBC haemolysis), severe jaundice, and death. ABO incompatibilities can be predicted from Table 6.4. Group AB individuals are 'universal recipients' as they have no circulating antibodies. Group O are 'universal donors' as they lack both A and B antigens. Alloantibodies against other antigens (e.g. Lewis, Kidd, Kelly, and Duffy) rarely cause clinically important transfusion reactions.

Table 6.3 Classification of anaemia according to underlying cause.[a]

Blood loss

Acute
- Trauma

Chronic
- Gastrointestinal lesions

Impaired red cell production

Defective DNA synthesis
- Deficiency of or impaired use of vitamin B_{12} or folic acid

Defective haemoglobin synthesis
- Deficient haem synthesis: iron deficiency
- Deficient globin synthesis: thalassaemias

Increased rate of red cell destruction (haemolytic)

Red cell membrane disorders
- Disorders of membrane cytoskeleton: spherocytosis, elliptocytosis
- Disorders of lipid synthesis: selective increase in membrane lecithin

Red cell enzyme deficiency
- Glycolytic enzymes: pyruvate kinase deficiency
- Enzymes of hexose monophosphate shunt: glucose-6-phosphate dehydrogenase (G6PD) deficiency

Disorders of haemoglobin synthesis
- Deficient globin synthesis: thalassaemias
- Structurally abnormal haemoglobin synthesis (haemoglobinopathies): sickle cell, unstable haemoglobin

Antibody-mediated
- Isohaemagglutinins: transfusion reactions
- Autoantibodies: idiopathic, drug-associated, systemic lupus erythematosus (SLE), malignancy

Mechanical trauma
- Microangiopathic haemolytic anaemias: thrombotic thrombocytopenic purpura (TTP), disseminated intravascular coagulation (DIC)

Infections
- Malaria

Chemical injury
- Lead poisoning

[a] From Robbins S, Cotran R, Kumar V. *Pathologic Basis of Disease*, 6th edn. Philadelphia: WB Saunders, 1996: 605.

Cross-matching

Before an emergency blood transfusion, the blood must be grouped (typed) and cross-matched. Grouping entails exposing the patient's RBC to serum known to contain antibodies against A and B antigens to determine the blood group or type. Rhesus typing is also performed by exposing the patient's RBC to anti-D antigen. Cross-matching is then carried out by combining donor RBC with recipient serum. This, in effect, mimics the intended transfusion. Cross-matching confirms ABO/Rhesus typing, detects antibodies to the other systems, and detects those present only in low titres. An alternative to cross-matching is screening, whereby the recipient's serum is added to RBC of known antigenic composition. This detects the non-ABO antibodies in the recip-

Table 6.4 The ABO blood group system[a]

Phenotype	Genotype	Antigen	Antibody in serum	Approximate proportion based on UK estimate
A	AA, AO	A	Anti-B	42%
B	BB, BO	B	Anti-A	8%
AB	AB	A, B	None	4%
O	OO	None[b]	Anti-A, Anti-B	47%

[a] Data obtained from Bray J, Cragg P, Macknight A, et al. *Lecture Notes in Human Physiology*, 3rd edn. Oxford: Blackwell Scientific, 1994: 333.
[b] Red cells of group O have the unmodified form of the H antigen on their surfaces.

ient's blood that are most likely to cause transfusion reactions. Screening is routinely carried out on all donor blood, but for a potential recipient it is safer to cross-match.

Acute blood loss

In acute hypovolaemic shock, there is no evidence that transfusion of whole blood is indicated. Group O negative red cell concentrate in combination with colloids and/or crystalloids can be administered if no cross-matched units are available. Compared with administration of whole blood, this minimises the transfer of anti-A and anti-B antibodies to the patient. If group O negative whole blood is administered, further transfusions should be of the same group until anti-A and anti-B titres are determined, as these antibodies can react with either the patient's own serum or a subsequent type-specific transfusion. Other products that are extracted from donated whole blood are shown in Figure 6.1. Blood products derived from donated whole blood not shown include human albumin solution (5% or 25%), coagulation concentrates (e.g. factor VIII), immunoglobulin (e.g. anti-D), and granulocyte concentrate.

Massive transfusion (defined as administration of blood products totalling greater than the patient's estimated blood volume in 24 hours) can result in microvascular haemorrhage due to dilutional thrombocytopenia or disseminated intravascular coagulation (DIC). Moderate deficiency of coagulation factors (in particular factors V and VIII) is common in this setting, but does not contribute to microvascular haemorrhage until levels are less than 20% of normal. During massive transfusion, haemostatic function should be monitored regularly and transfusion of platelets and fresh frozen plasma administered when appropriate. Appropriate tests include the International Normalised Ratio (INR), activated partial thromboplastin time (aPTT), platelet count, fibrin degradation products, and possibly thromboelastography.

HAEMOSTASIS

Haemostasis is the process of blood clot formation at the site of vessel injury. Normally, it is carefully regulated to occur rapidly and to remain localised in its effect. The clotting process is a dynamic, interdependent array of processes that are normally balanced to prevent both spontaneous haemorrhage and intravascular clotting. Abnormal bleeding or unphysiological thrombosis (i.e. thrombosis not required for haemostatic regulation) can occur when specific elements of these processes are deficient or dysfunctional.

The role of platelets

The platelet plays a pivotal role in haemostasis. Platelets are activated at the site of vascular injury to form a platelet plug that provides the initial haemostatic response. They also are involved in the clotting cascade, vasoconstriction

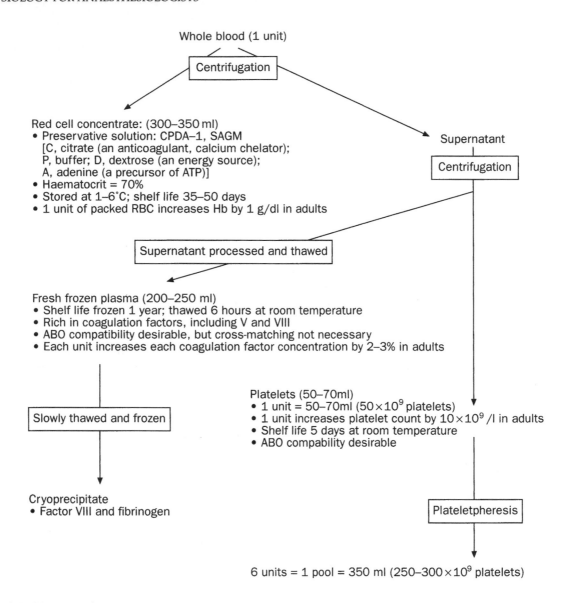

Figure 6.1 Blood products.

of the injured blood vessel, and tissue repair. Platelets are anucleate, granulated bodies derived from megakaryocytes in the bone marrow. The normal platelet count is $150–400 \times 10^9/l$ blood; the platelet half-life is 4 days.

Platelets are activated by exposed subendothelial collagen. Other weaker physiological stimuli include thrombin, adenosine diphosphate (ADP), and adrenaline. The plasma membrane of the platelet contains glycoproteins, which are receptors for platelet activation, adhesion, and aggregation. Glycoprotein GpIa–IIa, a platelet collagen receptor, is the most important in platelet activation. Platelet adhesion is primarily mediated by the binding of platelet surface receptor GpIb–IX–V complex to von Willebrand factor (vWF) in the subendothelial matrix. vWF, which is synthesised in megakaryocytes and endothelial cells, is also a carrier for factor VIII in the coagulation cascade. Platelet aggregation is mediated by GpIIb–IIIa, the most abundant receptor on the platelet surface. Following platelet activation, this receptor complex undergoes conformational change and binds immobilised fibrinogen. Fibrinogen is a divalent molecule that bridges the activated platelets.

Activated platelets secrete a variety of substances from their granules. Dense bodies store ADP and serotonin, which stimulate and recruit additional platelets, and calcium. Platelet-released serotonin normally causes vasodilation; however, it can induce vasoconstriction in the presence of damaged dysfunctional endothelium. The α granules contain numerous proteins, including fibronectin, thrombospondin, fibrinogen, vWF, and platelet factor 4. Fibronectin and thrombospondin are adhesive proteins that may reinforce and stabilise platelet aggregates. Fibrinogen released from the α granules provides a source of fibrinogen at sites of endothelial injury in addition to that present in plasma.

The platelet membrane contains phospholipids, primarily phosphatidylserine, which provide a surface for assembly of the enzyme complexes in the coagulation cascade on the platelet surface. The plasma membrane is also a source of arachidonic acid for synthesis of prostaglandins. Thromboxane A_2 (TxA_2) a prostaglandin metabolite, promotes vasoconstriction and further platelet activation.

Coagulation cascade and propagation of the clot

The central feature of the coagulation cascade is its sequential activation of a series of proenzymes or inactive precursor proteins (zymogens) to active enzymes. The activation of these zymogens (coagulation factors) results in stepwise amplification and conversion of soluble fibrinogen (factor I) to insoluble fibrin by the protease enzyme thrombin (factor IIa). The local generation of fibrin enmeshes and reinforces the platelet plug.

The coagulation factors are mostly globulins synthesised in the liver . The vitamin K-dependent procoagulants are factors II, VII, IX, and X. There are also two vitamin K-dependent anticoagulants: protein C and protein S (see below). Vitamin K is required for the synthesis of both of these, and Ca^{2+} is required for their activation.

The coagulation cascade consists of intrinsic and extrinsic pathways (Figure 6.2). These converge on the activation of factor X, which then activates the conversion of prothrombin to thrombin, the final enzyme of the cascade. Thrombin converts fibrinogen from a soluble plasma protein into insoluble fibrin. The intrinsic pathway is initiated by the exposure of blood to a negatively charged surface (such as glass in the aPTT clotting time). The extrinsic pathway is activated by tissue factor (TF) exposed at the site of injury or tissue factor-like material (thromboplastin, TPL).

Multicomponent complexes also play a major role in coagulation. These consist of the coagulation factor(s), cofactor proteins, calcium ions, and cellular membrane components (anionic phospholipid surfaces of platelets).

Extrinsic pathway

Vessel wall injury leads to expression of TF (tissue thromboplastin), which is not expressed on the normal intact endothelial cell surface. Tissue thromboplastin is the cofactor required for activation of factor VII. The TF–factor VIIa complex in turn activates factors X and IX. Factor IXa in complex with factor VIIIa also activates factor X. This dual pathway of factor X activation (i.e. directly and indirectly by activation of factor IX) is necessary because of the limited amount of TF generated in vivo.

When factor X is activated, the coagulation cascade proceeds as follows: factor V (also released from platelet α granules during platelet activation) is cleaved by thrombin to form activated factor V (factor Va) and binds factor Xa. Platelet factor V appears to be more important for assembly of the prothrombinase complex than circulating factor V.

Factor Xa linked to factor Va on the platelet phospholipid surface forms the prothrombinase complex, which converts prothrombin (factor II) to its activated form, thrombin (factor IIa). Thrombin converts fibrinogen to fibrin, which polymerises in the presence of factor XIIIa from

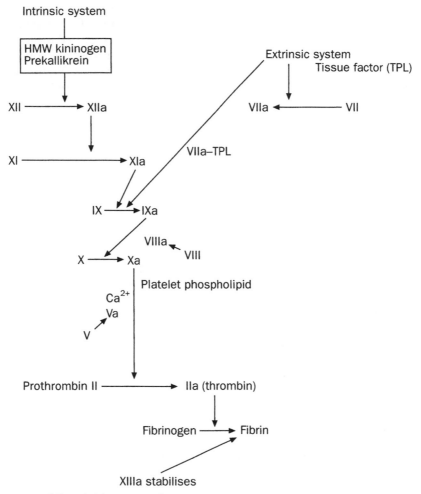

Figure 6.2 *Summary of the clotting cascade.*

its unstable to its stable form. A strong insoluble clot results.

Intrinsic pathway

The initial phase of the intrinsic or contact activation pathway consists of several plasma proteins – factor XII (Hageman factor), prekallikrein (Fletcher factor), and kininogen – which are activated by contact with negatively charged surfaces and which initiate the following sequence. Factor XIIa, in conjunction with high-molecular-weight kininogen (HMWK, Fitzgerald factor), activates factor XI (plasma thromboplastin antecedent), which in turn activates factor IX.

The remainder of the intrinsic system follows the common pathway involving factor V, prothrombin, and fibrinogen.

Control mechanisms and termination of clotting

The interaction of activated platelets with the coagulation cascade is potentially explosive, and if unchecked could lead to thrombosis, vascular inflammation, and tissue damage. Coagulation is therefore controlled by a number of mechanisms, such as dilution of procoagulants in flowing blood and removal of activated factors through the reticuloendothelial system, and by natural antithrombotics. These natural antithrombotics include antithrombin III and proteins C and S.

Antithrombin III (AT III) is a circulating plasma protease inhibitor. It inactivates many of the enzymes in the coagulation cascade, especially thrombin. The binding of endogenous or exogenous heparin to its binding site on AT III produces a conformational change in AT III that accelerates the inactivating process 1000- to 4000-fold.

As clot formation progresses, thrombin (factor IIa) binds to thrombomodulin (TM), an integral membrane protein on the endothelial cell surface. Binding of TM induces a conformational change in thrombin, which in turn acquires the ability to activate protein C. Activated protein C (APC), in association with protein S on phospholipid surfaces, proteolytically inactivates various coagulation factors.

The role of the endothelium

The endothelium plays a role in both the haemostatic response and the control and termination of the clotting process. Its role in the initiation of the clotting cascade and its interaction with platelets have already been described. The endothelium also acts to keep the process in check by a number of mechanisms.

Intact endothelial cells in proximity to disrupted endothelium release arachidonic acid from cell membrane phospholipids by phospholipase A_2. The enzyme cyclooxygenase-1 (COX-1) converts arachidonic acid into TxA_2 in platelets and prostacyclin (PGI_2) in endothelial cells. TxA_2 is a potent stimulator of platelet aggregation, causing vasoconstriction. PGI_2, in contrast, blocks platelet aggregation and antagonises TxA_2-mediated vasoconstriction. In this way, the intact endothelium, via PGI_2, maintains control of the coagulation process.

Low-dose aspirin irreversibly acetylates and inhibits COX-1. Since platelets cannot synthesise new COX-1, inhibition of TxA_2 is permanent for the life of the platelet. In contrast, endothelial cells can synthesise new COX-1, and greater doses are required to inhibit PGI_2 production. This is the mechanism that underlies the benefit of low-dose aspirin to patients with cardiovascular disease.

Nitric oxide (NO) is formed from L-arginine in endothelial cells, catalysed by the enzyme nitric oxide synthase (NOS). Acting through guanylate cyclase and cyctic guanosine monophosphate (cGMP), it causes vasodilatation and inhibits platelet adhesion and aggregation. NO is rapidly destroyed by haemoglobin and functions as another means by which the endothelium serves to regulate haemostasis.

Clot elimination and fibrinolysis

To restore vessel patency following haemostasis, the clot must be organized and removed by plasmin in conjunction with wound healing and tissue remodelling. Plasmin lyses both fibrin and fibrinogen with release of fibrinogen degradation products (FDPs). One such FDP is D-dimer, which consists of two D domains from adjacent fibrin monomers that have been cross-linked by activated factor VIII.

Plasmin is derived from its inactive precursor, plasminogen, by the action of thrombin and tissue-type plasminogen activator (tPA). The latter is a serine protease plasminogen activator secreted by vascular endothelial cells. Another form of tPA, urokinase-type plasminogen activator (uPA), is found in tears and saliva. Both tPA and uPA are inhibited by plasminogen activator inhibitors, while α_2 antiplasmin inhibits plasmin. Activated protein C inhibits these plasminogen activator inhibitors.

WHITE BLOOD CELLS (Table 6.5)

The white blood cell count is normally $4–11 \times 10^9/l$. These consist of polymorphonuclear leucocytes (neutrophils, basophils, and eosinophils), which have multilobular nuclei and cytoplasmic granules. Having a half-life of only 6 hours, over 100 billion neutrophils are produced each day. Neutrophils act mainly as phagocytes in acute inflammation. After 72 hours in the circulation, monocytes enter the tissues to function as macrophages. These include Kupffer cells in the liver, pulmonary alveolar macrophages, and microglia in the brain. Macrophages are activated by T lymphocytes. Eosinophils are numerous in the respiratory, lower urinary, and gastro-

Table 6.5 Differential white cell count, morphology, and function of white blood cells

White blood cell	Function	% of total	Morphology
Neutrophil	Phagocytosis in acute inflammation	40–75	Multilobar nucleus, granular cytoplasm
Lymphocyte	Cellular and humoral immunity	20–45	Monolobar nucleus, thin rim of cytoplasm
Monocyte	Precursor of tissue macrophage	2–10	Large irregular nucleus
Eosinophil	Parasitic infection, phagocytosis of antigen–antibody complexes; modulates the effect of histamine and leukotrienes in allergic reactions	1–6	Bilobar nucleus, large granules containing major basic protein
Basophil	Delayed hypersensitivity reaction	<1	Large irregular nucleus, containing heparin and histamine

intestinal tracts, where they probably play a role in mucosal immunity. Basophils express IgE on their cell surfaces and release histamine and heparin in immediate hypersensitivity reactions.

FURTHER READING

Bennett JS, Vilaire G. Exposure of platelet fibrinogen receptors by ADP and epinephrine. *J Clin Invest* 1979; **64**: 1393–401.

Bray J, Cragg P, Macknight A, et al. *Lecture Notes in Human Physiology*, 3rd edn. Oxford: Blackwell Scientific, 1994: 327–39.

Chasis JA, Mohandas N. Erythrocyte membrane deformability and stability: two distinct membrane properties that are independently regulated by skeletal protein associations. *J Cell Biol* 1986; **103**: 343–50.

Clarke RJ, Mayo G, Price P, Fitzgerald GA. Suppression of thromboxane A_2 but not of systemic prostacyclin by controlled-release aspirin. *N Engl J Med* 1991; **325**: 1137–41.

Edelberg JM, Pizzo SV. Lipoprotein (a) promotes plasmin inhibition by α_2-antiplasmin. *Biochem J* 1992; **286**: 79–84.

Ganong W. *Review of Medical Physiology*, 19th edn. Stamford, CT: Appleton and Lange, 1999: 508–20.

Goldstone J, Pollard B. *Handbook of Clinical Anaesthesia*. Edinburgh: Churchill Livingstone, 1996: 172–3.

Harrison P, Savidge GF, Cramer EM. The origin and physiological relevance of alpha-granule adhesive proteins. *Br J Haematol* 1990; **74**: 125–30.

Hoylaerts M, Rijken DC, Lijnen HR. Kinetics of the activation of plasminogen by human tissue plasminogen activator. Role of fibrin. *J Biol Chem* 1982; **257**: 2912–19.

Kroll MH, Schafer AI. Biochemical mechanisms of platelet activation. *Blood* 1989; **74**: 1181–95.

LaCelle PL, Weed RI. The contribution of normal and pathologic erythrocytes to blood rheology. *Prog Hematol* 1971; **7**: 1–31.

Marcum JA, McKenney JB, Rosenberg RD. Acceleration of thrombin–antithrombin complex formation in rat hindquarters via heparin-like molecules bound to the endothelium. *J Clin Invest* 1984; **74**: 341–50.

Mohandas N, Chasis JA. Red blood cell deformability, membrane material properties and shape: regulation by transmembrane, skeletal and cytosolic proteins and lipids. *Semin Hematol* 1993; **30**: 171–92.

Mohandas N, Evans E. Mechanical properties of the red cell membrane in relation to molecular structure and genetic defects. *Annu Rev Biophys Biomol Struct* 1994; **23**: 787–818.

Moncada S, Higgs A. The L-arginine–nitric oxide pathway. *N Engl J Med* 1993; **329**: 2002–12.

Mosesson MW. The roles of fibrinogen and fibrin in hemostasis and thrombosis. *Semin Hematol* 1992; **29**: 177–88.

Robbins S, Cotran R, Kumar V. *Pathologic Basis of Disease*, 6th edn. Philadelphia: WB Saunders, 1996.

Samis JA, Ramsey GD, Walker JB. Proteolytic processing of human coagulation factor IX by plasmin. *Blood* 2000; **95**: 943–51.

Savage B, Shattil SJ, Ruggeri ZM. Modulation of

platelet function through adhesion receptors: a dual role for glycoprotein IIb–IIIa (integrin $\alpha_{IIb}\beta_3$) mediated by fibrinogen and glycoprotein Ib–von Willebrand factor. *J Biol Chem* 1992; **267**: 11 300–6.

Savage B, Saldivar E, Ruggeri ZM. Initiation of platelet adhesion by arrest onto fibrinogen or translocation on von Willebrand factor. *Cell* 1996; **84**: 289–97.

Watson SP. Collagen receptor signaling in platelets and megakaryocytes. *Thromb Haemost* 1999; **82**: 365–76.

Weed RI. The importance of erythrocyte deformability. *Am J Med* 1970; **49**: 147–50.

Weiss L, Tavassoli M. Anatomic hazards to the passage of erythrocytes through the spleen. *Semin Hematol* 1970; **7**: 372–80.

Zeidel ML. Recent advances in water transport. *Semin Nephrol* 1998; 18: 167–77.

7

The endocrine system

William FM Wallace

DEFINITION AND SCOPE

Endocrine glands are distinguished from exocrine glands because they secrete within the body (endo) rather than out of the body (exo). The hormones that they secrete pass via the circulation to produce an effect by acting on target organs. This chapter considers the hormones most relevant to anaesthetic practice: insulin, thyroid hormones, hormones of the adrenal cortex and medulla, and parathormone. Within this framework, other hormones and influences are also considered, since the body's responses are always complex. Thus glucose metabolism during intensive care is influenced by such hormones as insulin, glucagon, cortisol, and thyroxine, as well as autonomic nerves and local factors in damaged tissues.

The next part of the chapter looks at the question, 'Why an endocrine system?', and at the end of the chapter the stress response is examined to illustrate the complex interactions of the endocrine, nervous, and cytokine systems. A notable example of such interactions is given by the sympathetic activating response, evoked in 'fight and flight' situations. Here the sympathetic nerves produce skin pallor, sweating, tremor, and tachycardia. At the same time, preganglionic sympathetic neurones activate the adrenal medulla to release large amounts of adrenaline and smaller amounts of noradrenaline and related hormones of the catecholamine family. Finally, if the response is prolonged, noradrenaline released as a neurotransmitter accumulates in the circulation to act together with the hormonal noradrenaline from the adrenal medulla – a neurotransmitter has become a hormone.

In recent decades, many other chemicals have been discovered, that add to the transmitter/hormonal cocktail in the circulation. Some are released and act on the releasing cell itself (autocrines) or on nearby cells (paracrines). Others are released from individual cells, particularly white blood cells, act locally, and also enter the circulation to act in many respects like hormones – the cytokines.

So, as usual in the body, there is local control where this is appropriate, and central control when the overall well-being of the body requires it. As indicated above, endocrine control is a vital part of overall control, and, not surprisingly, the brain is dominant. Hormonal effects are for the well-being of the brain and are ultimately controlled by it.

WHY AN ENDOCRINE SYSTEM?

Low-cost, low-speed control

As discussed above, the nervous and the endocrine systems are both control systems that release chemical transmitters to act on receptors in the target organs. The difference between the two systems is largely in speed and cost. A costly system in this context is one that is bulky and uses a lot of energy. The nervous system is high in speed and cost, while the endocrine system is low in both. Even within the nervous system, the reciprocity of speed and cost applies strongly. The fastest neurones are large and myelinated. They can convey an impulse from brain to big toe in about 0.04 s. Unmyelinated sympathetic fibres take 50–100 times as long. Bulk is related to cross-sectional area, which is proportional to radius squared. With the ratio of radii about 15 : 1, the cross-sectional area ratio is around 225 : 1 for large myelinated nerves versus small unmyelinated nerves.

An advantage of the endocrine system is that the bulk and cost of transmission are reduced to zero, since the transmitter is carried free of charge in the circulation. Of course, speed is correspondingly reduced, since the circulating time from capillaries in the endocrine gland to the heart and out to the capillaries of target organs is around 1 minute. Since the effect builds up as the hormone level rises in the circulation, the peak effect may be 10 minutes or more after the onset of secretion – some 15 000 times slower than the effect of the fastest nerves. The switch-off effect is also relatively slow. Many hormones, for example insulin and vasopressin (antidiuretic hormone, ADH), have a half-life of 5–10 minutes in the circulation. With a half-life of 10 minutes, concentration will halve each 10 minutes, falling to one-eighth in half an hour. So a hormone effect may take up to half an hour to disappear.

In general, somatic nerves produce effects (such as reflexively avoiding stumbling) in a fraction of a second, autonomic nerves produce effects within seconds and endocrine control produces effects within minutes that may last for minutes or hours.

Widespread selective control

Hormones can control organs throughout the body, provided the appropriate receptors are present and access is not limited at capillary level (as with the blood–brain barrier). Increasingly, hormones are being found to have multiple sites of action, which produce a package of coordinated effects that radically alter body function. For example, adrenaline favours a hyperdynamic state of the circulation, increased conductivity of the airways, speeding of skeletal muscle reflex responses, and dilation of the pupils, all of which help in the 'fight or flight' response.

A different person

The individual under the influence of adrenaline is thus in many respects a different person – able to run faster, fight more effectively, and move greater weights.

Another example, with a totally different timescale, is the effect of the sex hormones at puberty. Male sex hormones not only increase muscle strength but also affect behaviour, promoting aggressiveness and sexual activity – distinguishing the men from the boys. Female sex hormones lead to the physical and psychological variations of the menstrual cycle, with a variety of effects favouring conception and the onset of pregnancy.

Following fertilisation, the hormonal cocktail of pregnancy favours the incubation and subsequent delivery of the baby, impairing physical activity in a variety of ways. The hormone relaxin favours delivery through the more flexible pelvis, but can make walking quite uncomfortable. It is as though certain situations can press certain buttons that change the person via the endocrine system to adapt to new circumstances.

Figure 7.1 is a light-hearted attempt to indicate this 'different person' effect of the endocrine system. The stress response at the end of this chapter is a more serious example of change of body function to meet the needs of patients undergoing major surgery or suffering from severe trauma in the intensive care unit. It is as though endocrine buttons are pressed in ways that are predictable and relevant to perioperative management.

INSULIN

Normal secretion and routine use by diabetics

Although insulin is often thought of as the hormone that keeps down blood glucose, it fits the concept of a substance that comprehensively changes body function in that it leads to the nutrient assimilation state. This state is characterised by entry of the great bulk of absorbed

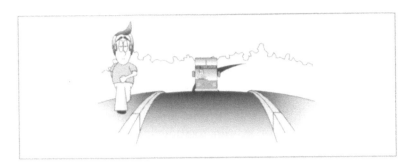

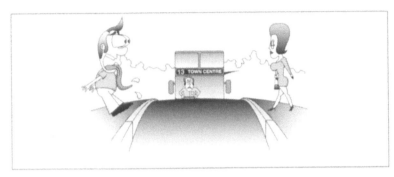

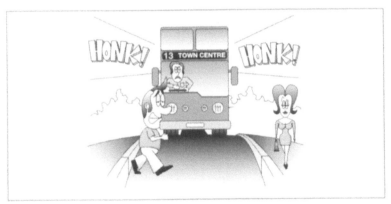

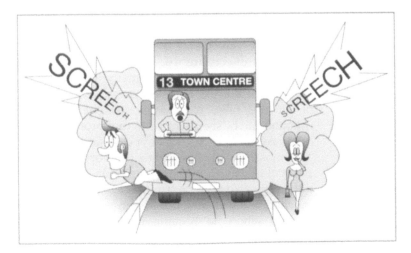

Figure 7.1 *This sets the scene for the concept that we become different sorts of people as our endocrine activities change. In the top panel, the bus driver and pedestrian are in the alert day-time state typical of our routine waking hours. In the second panel, the pedestrian (male) notices an attractive female friend – an event of significance because of the long-term effects of different sex hormones.*
In the next panel, the pedestrian rushes across the road without noticing the bus. In this and the bottom panel virtually instanta-neous accident-avoiding actions prevent disaster with the aid of the sympathetic nervous system and its catecholamines. In the next few minutes, both driver and pedestrian will experience the effects of the endocrine cate-cholamine surge and will be rather shaken people with palpi-tations, tremor, pallor, and per-haps sweating.

nutrients into body stores – particularly carbo-hydrates into the glycogen stores of skeletal muscle and the liver, fat into the subcutaneous fat stores, and amino acids and potassium into skeletal muscle. Overall, this is an anabolic state, building up muscle bulk and filling tissue ener-gy stores. The state includes vascular changes and (particularly when associated with a major meal after major physical exertion) marked lethargy and drowsiness. Hormones other than insulin are probably involved, with circulating gut hormones promoting drowsiness.

The insulin-controlled nutrient assimilation state can be regarded as the fourth stage of nutrition – following ingestion, digestion, and absorption. It has long been known that insulin secretion is greater after oral than intravenous administration of a given amount of glucose. This is because nervous and particularly gut hormonal activity during ingestion and early digestion stimulate insulin secretion, which is maintained by the rising blood levels of the absorbed substances, particularly glucose. In this way, excessive build-up of nutrients (which would exceed the renal threshold and be lost in the urine) is prevented, because insulin levels rise synchronously with nutrient levels and the nutrients flow smoothly from the blood into the stores of the hepatocytes, adiposites, and skele-tal muscle. Physical exercise has a useful effect on this. It has been shown that the glycogen granules of skeletal muscle fill most efficiently shortly after vigorous exercise. Insulin require-ments (including for diabetics) are reduced by exercise. It is important that diabetics exercise and it is important that exercising diabetics take care to avoid a dangerous fall in blood glucose by adjusting nutrient intake upwards and insulin intake downwards. The article by Kjeldy in the further reading at the end of this chapter gives a fascinating account of a general practi-tioner with diabetes mellitus who successfully completed a marathon.

The normal daily variations in blood insulin are illustrated in Figure 7.2a, showing that secre-tion of insulin is related in time and amount to the timing and size of the meal. It is interesting to compare this with the evolution of insulin therapy. For many years, most patients were treated with a single injection at the beginning of the day (Figure 7.2b). This led to a steady level of circulating insulin, rather than the required fluctuating level. So blood glucose fluc-tuated more than normal, with hyperglycaemia and glycosuria alternating with hypoglycaemia, with its threat of coma and death. Early in the history of insulin treatment, some meticulous patients with a scientific bent used more fre-quent injections, related to meals and informed by regular testing of urine (blood testing was not then available to patients). These patients often maintained excellent health and led the way to the present policy of a regime as close as possible to the normal pattern (Figure 7.2a). Insulin is now seen as part of the menu for a meal, and a dose for the meal is computed and administered. Frequent blood glucose levels can be determined by patients, who aim to keep the blood glucose at a level that suits them. In gen-eral, levels are kept a little higher than normal, since occasional glycosuria is better than occa-sional hypoglycaemia.

Anaesthetic applications

The trainee anaesthetist needs to be familiar with the features of hypoglycaemia, ketoacido-sis (although major problems are managed by diabetologists), and perioperative management.

Hypoglycaemia

This is the usual cause of abrupt impairment of consciousness in the diabetic patient. The attacks are dangerous, and sometimes fatal. They have direct and compensatory features. The direct effects are due to impaired cerebral metabolism. Brain cells normally depend on bloodborne glucose for energy, and, as the level of glucose falls, progressive loss of cerebral function can be seen, similar to that produced by other depressants such as hypoxia and alcohol. The most sensitive cells are the cortical cells, particularly those in the frontal area concerned with critical decisions. Colleagues of a distin-guished medical diabetic diagnosed hypogly-caemia when he became unreasonable at a committee meeting. Patients may complain of

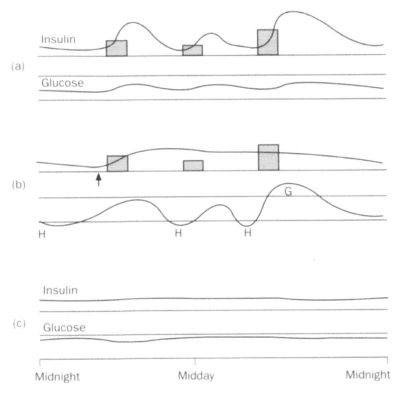

Figure 7.2 *(a) Fluctuating insulin (above) and glucose (below) levels in the blood over a 24-hour period. The marked peaks in insulin and lesser peaks in glucose are related to the three meals taken. After the meal, the individual is biochemically in the assimilative state, with absorbed nutrients flowing into stores in an orderly way. (b) The very different pattern with someone whose sole source of insulin is a daily injection (arrow). On three occasions, blood glucose falls below normal into the hypoglycaemic zone (H). On one occasion, it exceeds the renal threshold for glycosuria (G). The aim of modern treatment is to have a pattern as close as possible to (a). (c) The situation perioperatively, where, hopefully, a constant infusion of glucose and insulin provides acceptable glucose levels throughout.*

feeling 'fuzzy' or 'woozy' and, again, companions may notice mildly inappropriate behaviour. In this state, driving would be dangerous, as with alcohol. Around this stage, compensatory responses are seen. Although hormones such as glucagon, cortisol, and growth hormone are raised, the most striking features are due to reflex sympathetic nervous system activity, with adrenaline from the adrenal medulla – skin pallor, sweating, tremor, and a hyperdynamic circulation (tachycardia plus a high pulse pressure). Many patients treat the 'hypo' appropriately with something sweet by mouth. However, perversely, the confused state of mind may prevent the patient from recognising the

problem. Friends may have to work hard to get the patient to ingest the appropriate glucose, chocolate, etc. Fortunately, the reflex (initiated by hypothalamic glucose sensors) includes vagal activity so that the glucose is absorbed rapidly. The risk of death is particularly great when the patient is alone or asleep, when friends cannot help.

Ketoacidosis

This arises from a severe deficiency of insulin action. The cause may be inadequate secretion, insulin resistance, or antagonism by the sympathetic nervous system, and hormones such as glucagon and cortisol. Ketoacidosis is often provoked in the treated diabetic by stresses such as infections, which increase insulin requirements. Sometimes the patient who is unable to eat normally may cut down on insulin inappropriately, fearing hypoglycaemia.

In the absence of insulin, energy metabolism is seriously deranged. Substrates in the blood increases because insulin is no longer keeping them in storage sites. Excess lipid metabolism in particular leads to release of ketoacids. The result is a torrent of hydrogen ions – the ultimate metabolic acidosis, whereby grossly abnormal metabolism leads directly to the excess hydrogen ions. The result is a drop in blood pH, in severe cases below 7.0.

The body tries to deal with the excess hydrogen ions in three ways. First, buffering takes place using the body's proteins and bicarbonate. The bicarbonate reserves are rapidly depleted and fall to half normal in moderately severe cases, and much lower in severe cases. Second, renal excretion of hydrogen ions increases. The urinary pH falls to its lower limit of around 4–5. This is accompanied by increased generation of bicarbonate, which, however, cannot keep pace with destruction due to buffering. Urinary synthesis and excretion of ammonia increase so that more hydrogen ions are excreted without further depressing urinary pH. Third, respiratory compensation occurs – the low pH stimulates ventilation; this leads to loss of carbon dioxide and a compensating respiratory alkalosis. However, in the absence of insulin, these compensating mechanisms merely slow fatal accumulation of hydrogen ions.

Ketoacidosis stimulates the chemoreceptor trigger zone in the brainstem to cause vomiting. Any benefit from loss of hydrogen ions is more than counterbalanced by fluid loss. Fluid loss is also favoured by osmotic diuresis due to the severe hyperglycaemia that accompanies the ketoacidosis. The extracellular fluid volume falls, and this leads to peripheral circulatory failure.

Treatment of ketoacidosis essentially requires insulin and intravenous normal saline. Insulin favours normal storage of glucose, etc., in the liver and other tissues, reducing blood glucose and turning off the torrent of hydrogen ions so that compensatory mechanisms can begin to return the pH to normal. Saline restores extracellular fluid volume and hence blood volume and circulation.

Perioperative management

Problems are less severe for diabetics on diet alone, or diet combined with oral drugs, but those requiring insulin face a major challenge during surgery and anaesthesia. Interruption of normal nutrition is accompanied by the response to physical stress, which includes hormonal effects antagonising insulin. During the perioperative period, such patients require frequent measurements of blood sugar level. These guide management, which usually consists of a combination of intravenous glucose and insulin (Figure 7.2c). The glucose avoids the risk of hypoglycaemia and the intravenous insulin is adjusted regularly in line with the blood glucose level. Because of the fairly intensive management thus required, the diabetic patient should be put first on an elective operation list to minimise delays.

THYROID HORMONES

The hormones considered here are thyroxine (T_4) and triiodothyronine (T_3). The other hormone of the thyroid – (thyro)calcitonin – plays a minor role in calcium homeostasis. The numbers in T_3 and T_4 refer to the iodine atoms attached to the thyronine structure of these hormones, which consists of two tyrosine units. The hormones are synthesised in the follicles of the thyroid gland in a matrix of the large protein molecule thyroglobulin. They have similar effects on thyroid receptors, but T_4 is much more highly bound to circulating plasma proteins, is released more slowly, and has a much slower onset and offset of action.

The influence of the thyroid hormones is largely on mitochondria, where they accelerate activity, increasing substrate use, oxygen uptake, carbon dioxide and heat production, and the availability of cellular energy in the form of adenosine triphosphate (ATP). The hormones enter the cell and act via the nucleus to increase synthesis of mitochondrial enzymes. The overall action in normal people can be appreciated by comparing people with overactive and underactive thyroid glands – thyrotoxicosis and myxoedema respectively.

In thyrotoxicosis, the effects mirror those described above on mitochondria. Increased substrate use leads to depletion of body tissues, particularly fat stores, so that the patient loses weight and subcutaneous fat is diminished. The body responds to the loss of weight by an increase in appetite. Alimentary tract activity increases and there is an increased frequency of defecation. Increased oxygen consumption and increased carbon dioxide production are associated with increased pulmonary ventilation, and the patient may interpret this as dyspnoea. Increased heat production leads to reflex heat-dissipating responses – increased peripheral blood flow and a hyperdynamic circulation with raised pulse pressure and increased sweating. Overall, these effects make the patient feel uncomfortably warm in a thermoneutral environment (where normal people feel most comfortable) – heat intolerance. The patient prefers a cooler environment and may open windows, to the discomfort of others. The situation is quite like that of the pregnant woman who also has an increased metabolic rate due to the superimposed fetal tissues, and who also is heat-intolerant.

The increased energy available to most tissues (the brain is a notable exception) tends to increase their function. An example of this is the pacemaker tissue of the heart. The intrinsic heart rate (the rate when extrinsic influences such as sympathetic and parasympathetic nerves are removed) increases in thyrotoxicosis. With most body tissues in overdrive, there are multiple reasons for increased organ activity. Thus the heart rate is intrinsically increased as mentioned above. It appears also to be increased by an increased intrinsic activity of sympathetic nerves, and it is also reflexively increased to maintain the increased cardiac output demanded by overactive tissues and increased heat production. Another example is the gut, which is stimulated by increased food intake and by increased autonomic activity – in this case mainly parasympathetic.

The overall effect is to produce a thin, sweating, tremulous (increased sympathetic activity), anxious, and uncomfortable patient, because the extra energy is inappropriate to the patient's needs and just produces unwanted effects.

In contrast, the patient with myxoedema is short of energy in many tissues, feeling lethargic, weak, and cold. Cardiac activity is depressed, peripheral circulation is poor, food intake and gut activity decrease with consequent constipation, and the low level of sympathetic activity is associated with drowsiness and even coma.

Thus the normal activity of the thyroid gland is needed for the normal everyday basal state upon which all other activity is built. What is less clear is why we have the ability to vary thyroid activity (via the hypothalamus, thyrotropin-releasing hormone, and pituitary thyroid-stimulating hormone). Increased activity would seem to be beneficial in cold environments, but there is little evidence that this is of much importance in practice. Since the effects of both inadequate available energy and excessive available energy lead to severe general malfunction (two different types of inappropriate different person), it seems that in some way the thyroid is controlled to deliver precisely the right amount of energy in a variety of circumstances.

Anaesthetic applications

These concern the risks of hyper- and hypothyroidism. Overactivity of the thyroid can lead to two major crises: cardiac failure and hyperthermia. This is because the increased cardiac drive, with tachycardia and increased cardiac output, may act in conjunction with otherwise insignificant cardiac weakness or ischaemia to precipitate dysrhythmia, notably atrial fibrillation, or cardiac failure. The increased basal metabolic rate tends to raise basal core temperature and hence increases the risk of an abnormal rise.

Underactivity carries a mirror-image risk of hypothermia, but paradoxically cardiac failure is also a problem here because prolonged hypothyroidism damages cardiac muscle. Because of the chronic depression of cerebral activity, these patients may be unusually sensitive to drugs that have a similar depressant activity on the brain.

ADRENAL CORTEX

The adrenal cortex secretes two major groups of hormones and one minor group. The major groups are the glucocorticoids, with cortisol as the main representative, and the mineralocorticoids, with aldosterone as the main representative. The minor group comprises androgens. These produce general effects of puberty in both sexes, such as axillary and pubic hair, and will not be considered further. The two major hormones – cortisol and aldosterone – will now be considered in turn.

Cortisol

This hormone provides another very good example of the different person effect of a hormone. Someone with a high normal level of cortisol has a very different bodily function as compared with someone with a low normal level, and someone with the much higher level of cortisol associated with severe physical stress is very different again. In very simple terms, the normal person with a low normal level is fit to lie asleep in bed, but is not in a position to deal with the stresses of everyday life, including maintaining the upright posture without light-headedness. The person with a moderate to high level is fit for everyday life (the level will rise with moderate stress such as strenuous exercise). The person with the much higher level of cortisol is fit to fight successfully for survival after a serious car crash.

Cortisol's effects are often described, rather negatively, as catabolic. It is true that the higher the level of cortisol, the faster are body tissues being broken down (catabolised). From this point of view, the normal low nocturnal level of cortisol avoids this and allows rebuilding of tissues (anabolism). However, a more positive way of describing the same effect is to regard cortisol

as the hormone that prevents acute circulatory failure – assuming other neuroendocrine functions and body fluids to be normal.

The patient with adrenal failure gives an example of this. On attempting to get up in the morning and go about normal activities, the patient feels seriously weak, and is forced back into the lying-down position by light-headedness, nausea, and vomiting – rather like someone in the acute phase of food poisoning. At the top end of the stress spectrum, the anaesthetist will find that a patient in intensive care after very major surgery or severe trauma will show falling blood pressure and other features of shock if the body is not producing the high levels of cortisol needed in this situation.

Figure 7.3 shows the pattern of cortisol levels to be seen in someone living a normal life who is doubly unfortunate. This person breaks a leg at point A and is just recovering from this when, about a week later at point B, a much more serious injury leads to prolonged hospitalization. At the beginning of the graph, the days are marked by the normal circadian (or diurnal) rhythm of cortisol. In general, the level is high during the day and declines to a minimum around the middle of the sleeping period. With the lesser injury (A), the circadian rhythm is lost and replaced by a surge lasting several days, while with the more serious injury (B), the surge reaches higher levels and lasts much longer.

How does all this fit in with cortisol's classification as a glucocorticoid? And with other effects, such as suppressing inflammation and immune responses? The term 'glucocorticoid' arose because one of the clear effects of cortisol is to raise the blood glucose level. It does this at least partly by converting non-glucose substrates, particularly amino acids, into 'new' glucose (gluconeogenesis) – as opposed to releasing 'old' glucose from glycogen stores. This breakdown of amino acids removes them from the pool available for protein synthesis and repair, and this leads to the muscle wasting of catabolism. In addition, it greatly reduces synthesis of the new proteins involved in immune responses and inflammation. This would explain, again at least in part, the anti-inflammatory and immuno-supprevise effects.

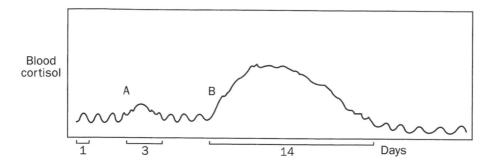

Figure 7.3 *An individual's blood cortisol levels are shown during a month in which a minor and a major injury occur. At the beginning and end of the month, the normal circadian rhythm of cortisol is seen, with the troughs around the middle of the sleeping period. At A, a minor injury leads to a cortisol surge lasting about 3 days. At B, a major injury leads to a much more pronounced and prolonged surge.*

In addition to its glucocorticoid actions, cortisol also possesses mineralocorticoid actions. At high levels of cortisol, these become marked. These effects are similar to and augment the actions of aldosterone (to be considered later).

Meanwhile, let us look at several cortisol disturbances that the trainee anaesthetist may encounter.

Cortisol suppression from steroid therapy

This potentially applies to all patients treated with exogenous steroids for weeks, months, or years. These steroids, given to suppress inflammation in such conditions as bronchial asthma and rheumatoid arthritis, include prednisone, and are in fact examples of synthetic pharmaceutical variations of cortisol. They are essentially glucocorticoids with the mineralocorticoid effects reduced as far as possible. Figure 7.4 illustrates why this large group of patients is liable to suffer from a form of adrenal cortical failure so that they cannot respond adequately to sudden stress such as trauma.

In the upper left of the diagram, the normal situation is shown, with hypothalamic corticotrophin-releasing hormone (CRH) (which passes along the pituitary portal vessels) controlling the circadian cortisol rhythm via adrenocorticotrophic hormone (ACTH). When severe trauma strikes (involving profound stimulation of pain pathways, upper right), ACTH

and cortisol respond with a great surge. In contrast, the patient who has received a course of endogenous steroid with its suppressing negative feedback on the pituitary cannot produce the surge, because both the relevant anterior pituitary and adrenal cortical cells have undergone disuse atrophy. So the only way in which the necessary surge can be achieved is by exogenous administration to the patient. The aim is to reproduce the extent and duration of the surge that would be normally expected. This may involve days or weeks of high-dosage steroid. Although in theory this may suppress healing and responses to infection, the priority is to prevent the fatal circulatory failure which would otherwise occur.

Adverse effects of steroid therapy

As well as the adrenal suppression mentioned above, patients on prolonged steroid therapy are liable to suffer from direct adverse effects. These are related particularly to excessive gluconeogenesis and excessive mineralocorticoid effects.

Excessive gluconeogenesis changes the amino acid–glucose balance in favour of glucose. There is an excess of glucose and a deficiency of amino acids. The excess glucose leads to a moderately increased circulating glucose level, and if the patient should suffer from diabetes mellitus then this complicates stabilisation. When the increased glucocorticoid activity is associated

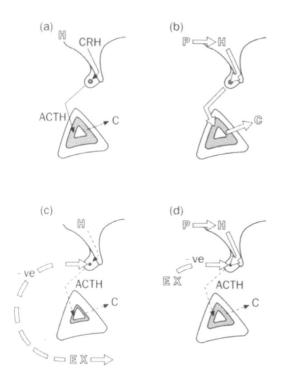

Figure 7.4 *The hypothalamic–pituitary–adrenal response to stress normally (a, b) and in someone with prolonged exogenous glucocorticoid ('steroid') treatment (c,d). On the left is the pre-stress situation with the basal hypothalamic stimulation. On the right is the response to severe physical stress which activates pain inputs (P), etc. In the lower diagrams the powerful negative feedback of exogenous steroid (E) has led to atrophy at pituitary and adrenal cortical level so there is no response to the stress signal. (ACTH, adrenocorticotrophic hormone; CRH, corticotrophin-releasing hormone.)*

with major stress, this glucose would be related to increased metabolism to provide energy for the lifesaving activities. However, if the glucose is not being utilised in this way, it tends to be laid down in fat, which contributes to the rounded facial appearance and weight gain.

The deficiency of amino acids produces catabolic effects. Muscles lose bulk and consequently strength. The immune system is depressed. Sometimes this is the purpose of the treatment, but in any case it weakens the patient's resist-

ance to infection. A particularly serious problem is loss of the protein collagen fibres that contribute significantly to bone strength. As a result, bone strength is compromised and fractures occur more readily. Collapse of vertebral bodies is a particularly distressing problem.

The increased mineralocorticoid action favours retention of salt and water. This favours an increase in arterial blood pressure and probably contributes to the facial rounding.

ADRENAL MEDULLA

The adrenal medulla can reasonably be regarded as part of the sympathetic nervous system, since it is usually activated along with sympathetic motor nerves and its hormonal output mimics sympathetic activity in many ways. It thus provides augmentation of sympathetic responses through the relatively economical but slow endocrine route compared with the faster and more focused nervous route, which is more expensive to the body in terms of space taken up and metabolic needs. The predominant hormone released is adrenaline, and this hormone is particularly suited to augment the sympathetic response to strenuous exercise and severe stress. Adrenaline, through its β effects, favours a hyperdynamic circulation and high metabolic rate, with cardiac inotropic and chronotropic effects, vaso- and bronchodilation, and mobilisation of glucose. In contrast, noradrenaline, a leading 'minority' secretion of the adrenal medulla, through its dominant α effects, favours vasoconstriction, hypertension (systolic and diastolic), and reflex bradycardia in response to the hypertension.

Anaesthetic applications

Anaesthetic practice is related to the adrenal medulla in two major situations. First, pharmaceutical analogues of adrenaline are used to support a circulation that is judged inadequate in the circumstances. Thus such treatment may be helpful in the perioperative period to augment oxygen delivery to tissues by a modest but critical increase in cardiac output.

Second, and relatively rarely, application of adrenal physiology is crucial in the perioperative period for patients undergoing surgery of the adrenals or related tissue. Adrenal tumours may secrete mainly adrenaline, mainly noradrenaline, or a combination of these and other hormones. The clinical situation often points to the diagnosis. Intermittent attacks or constant presence of hyperdynamic circulation (tachycardia with a wide pulse pressure) suggest predominant adrenaline secretion. Interestingly, the effects of constant release of adrenaline can mimic thyrotoxicosis, with tremor, heat intolerance, and sweating added to the hyperdynamic circulation. Hypertension with systolic and diastolic pressures raised in parallel suggest predominant noradrenaline secretion. Detailed biochemical studies are needed to confirm the hormone or hormones involved.

As usual, the aim in the perioperative period is to anticipate problems. Thus α blockade is required to control the effects of sudden release of noradrenaline (e.g. during surgery), while β blockade is indicated where adrenaline is the main hormone produced by the overactive gland.

PARATHORMONE

As the major hormone regulating blood calcium, parathormone (parathyroid hormone, PTH) is of particular significance in relation to neuromuscular excitability. It regulates this by regulating extracellular ionised calcium.

First, it is useful to consider the components of total blood calcium. About half the normal total is bound, mainly to plasma proteins. This calcium is not involved in neuromuscular excitability. The other major component is free ionised calcium. This is the component of physiological significance for excitability. Although other important functions, including blood clotting, depend on ionised calcium, changes in excitability are by far the commonest manifestations of abnormal levels (high or low) of this ion.

Both bound and ionised calcium vary independently, so it is usual to measure the main binder – albumin – at the same time. Figure 7.5 shows why this is necessary. For example in (b), when the protein is low and the ionised calcium normal, the total calcium is low. Correction for the low protein shows that there is no need to investigate calcium balance further. In contrast, (c) requires investigation of hypercalcaemia. In practice, increased protein levels (d, e) are rare. We shall now consider the effects of hypo- and hypercalcaemia.

Effects of disordered ionised extracellular calcium levels

The ionised calcium level in the blood is the same as that in the interstitial fluid, and this is why it is so important. It represents the level in both intra- and extravascular components of the extracellular fluid, and the level in cerebrospinal fluid is very similar. The excitable tissues – nerves and muscles – are bathed in this fluid (Figure 7.6), and its calcium ions profoundly influence excitability. Since excitability is produced by sudden influx of extracellular sodium ions, it is reasonable to conclude that extracellular calcium ions alter the configuration of the cell membrane protein constituting sodium channels. The effect is that low extracellular calcium favours opening of sodium channels and hyperexcitability (tetany) while high extracellular calcium depresses excitability.

These effects apply to sensory, motor, and cerebral neurones. So, in hypocalcaemic tetany, sensory nerves are hyperexcitable (paraesthesiae), motor nerves are hyperexcitable (muscle spasms), and cerebral neruones are hyperexcitable (increased risk of epilepsy).

With hypercalcaemia, all of these neurones are less active than normal, leading to weakness and lethargy.

Control and actions of parathormone

Like the nerves whose function they control, the parathyroid glands are stimulated by an environment low in calcium ions, and the hormone that they release raises the level of calcium ions. This is a very simple negative-feedback loop: low calcium triggers release of PTH, which

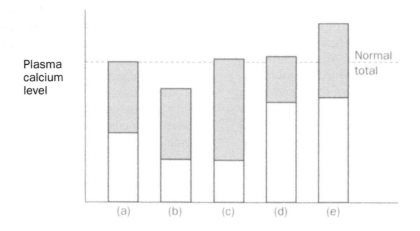

Figure 7.5 *Components of the total plasma calcium – protein-bound (clear rectangles) and free ionised (hatched rectangles). Compared with the normal situation (a), (b) shows normocalcaemia (i.e. a normal ionised level) which is recorded as a low total calcium (hypocalcaemia); (c) shows hypercalcaemia masquerading as normocalcaemia, (d) hypocalcaemia with a normal total, and (e) normocalcaemia masquerading as hypercalcaemia.*

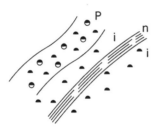

Figure 7.6 *On the upper left is a capillary with its plasma (P) containing a mixture of free (black semicircles) and bound (circles) calcium. Only the free calcium equilibrates with the interstitial fluid (i) which bathes the nerve (n).*

negates the low calcium. The main actions of PTH are threefold, and fit together logically.

First, the hormone releases calcium ions from the immense store of calcium in bone. Osteoclasts are stimulated, and these break down adjoining bone matrix to release calcium and phosphate ions. Following the laws of mass action, the product of calcium and phosphate concentrations is limited, so a raised phosphate

level opposes an increase in the calcium level. Therefore, second, it is appropriate that PTH increases phosphate excretion in the urine (phosphaturia). It does this by depressing reabsorption of phosphate from the filtrate. This effect is one reason why hyperparathyroidism favours deposition of calcium phosphate stones in the urinary tract (the other reason is that the hypercalcaemia of hyperparathyroidism leads to increased filtration and excess calcium also in the urine). With this loss of calcium from the bones via the urine, it is logical that, third, PTH increases activation of vitamin D. It does this by converting 25-hydroxycholecalciferol into 1,25-dihydroxycholecalciferol. The activated vitamin D then increases calcium absorption in the duodenum, restoring bone mineralisation and completing the negative-feedback loop that maintains bone mineralisation.

THE RESPONSE TO PHYSICAL STRESS

For many years, people have been aware of a recognisable changed bodily state in the severely ill due to severe trauma or extensive burns.

Many terms have been used: metabolic response to trauma, insulin resistance, catabolic state, hypermetabolic state, ebb phase, acute phase, negative nitrogen and potassium balance, and positive sodium and water balance. If the patient recovers, other terms come into play: anabolic state, flow phase, recovery phase, and positive nitrogen balance. Many of these effects are due to a cortisol surge and this has been discussed earlier in the section.

However, the response involves much more than cortisol – it includes many other hormones, autonomic nervous responses, and cytokines of the inflammatory response. Figure 7.7 indicates some of the components of this immensely complicated response, and some aspects will now be considered.

A blend of chemicals

The stress response is an example of how the various stimulating systems – nervous, endocrine, and cytokine – all acting through chemicals that stimulate or inhibit receptors on target organs – work together to produce effects that, in general, favour recovery.

Injury reduces blood volume in many ways: by external and internal haemorrhage, by loss of circulating fluid into areas of oedema, and sometimes by vomiting. These effects tend to cause circulatory failure. This is combated by a blend of sympathetic nervous activity (vasoconstriction in non-essential areas, and tachycardia) and endocrine activity (cortisol, as previously mentioned via its mineralocorticoid effects, aldosterone, the main mineralocorticoid, antidiuretic hormone/vasopressin by its water retention and also vasoconstricting effects).

All such responses consume energy, and Figure 7.7 indicates that a successful response must be fuelled with energy derived from substrate reserves – hence the vulnerability of the severely malnourished individual.

A graded response

Figure 7.8 indicates this concept. The level of stress is indicated on the horizontal axis in gen-

eral terms, and, for full-thickness burns, more precisely as the percentage of body surface affected. The response increases with the severity of the stress and then levels off – presumably a maximal response has been achieved and beyond this point survival is increasingly unlikely.

It has been noted that young, physically very fit individuals recover remarkably quickly from quite severe trauma, and a better-than-average stress response with excellent body reserves, particularly of protein, seems the likely explanation (Figure 7.8a). In contrast, the frail elderly or malnourished person is unable to produce much response and succumbs to relatively minor stress (Figure 7.8c).

A complexly variable response

Severe stress can produce a variety of complex injuries to the various body systems. Some trauma produces severe haemorrhage with relatively little general damage to body tissues. Burns lead to extensive damage and production of toxic produces, with more loss of body fluids and plasma than of red blood cells. Infections may act mainly by production of toxins. Inflammation may build up rapidly with time. Thus the input signals in Figure 7.7, particularly those via specific receptors, will vary widely. Similarly, the output will vary, with baroreceptor responses prominent where haemorrhage is the dominant problem. The time course of the response will also vary widely. Apart from the obviously longer response to massive stress, continuing infection and inflammation may prolong effects related to cytokines.

A largely beneficial response

Clearly, specific responses (e.g. to loss of blood) are vital, and in general the metabolic response is also essential (as shown by its potentially fatal absence in adrenal cortical failure). Since the response consumes so much of the body's reserves, it has been questioned whether it is sometimes greater than necessary. It has been suggested that effective pain relief can reduce

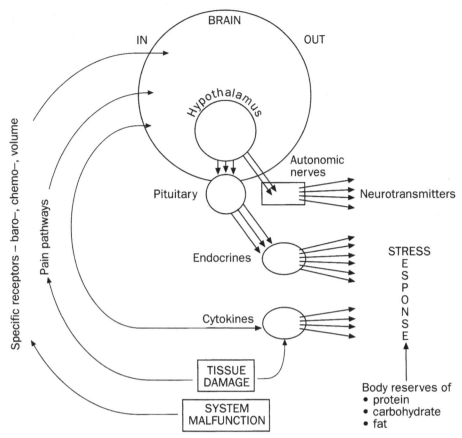

Figure 7.7 *A complex diagram indicating the complex body response to life-threatening injury and tissue damage. With all of these responses working and with adequate body reserves, the person has a good chance of surviving.*

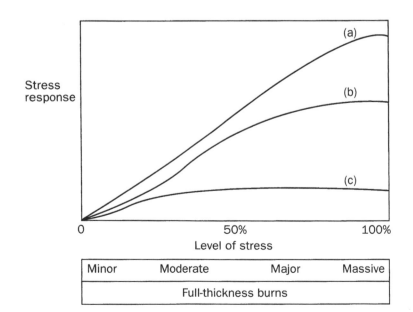

Figure 7.8 *A simple diagram, condensing the complex pattern of Figure 7.7 into a single 'stress response'. Examples of different levels of stress are shown. The average healthy adult, represented by (b), is likely to survive up to the beginning of the massive stress zone. An exceptionally fit young person (a) can survive greater stress and recover more quickly. A frail elderly person (c) will succumb to mild/moderate stress.*

the response somewhat without affecting survival. However, many attempts to manipulate the response and block it in various ways have produced little evidence of benefit. In general, prompt attention to specific problems (fluid balance, oxygen delivery, fractures, and damaged vessels and organs) acts at the source of the problem by reducing the level of stress. In contrast, when multiple complications lead to accumulation of toxic products and high levels of various cytokines, the syndromes of toxic shock and multiple organ failure frequently lead to death.

FURTHER READING

British Journal of Anaesthesia (Postgraduate Educational Issue). Endocrine and Metabolic Disorders in Anaesthesia and Intensive Care. *Br J Anaesth* 2000; **85**: 1–117.

Kjeldby B. Running the New York marathon with diabetes. *BMJ* 1997; **314**: 1053–4.

8

Renal physiology

CV Elzo Kraemer

INTRODUCTION

The kidneys are a pair of bean-shaped organs lying in the retroperitoneal space. The upper pole of each kidney is found opposite the 12th thoracic vertebra, while the lower pole lies opposite the 3rd lumbar vertebra. In humans, the kidneys weigh 150–170 g each and are about 11–13 cm in length. Approximately 180 l of glomerular filtrate is produced each day, 99% of which is reabsorbed. The nephron, the functional unit of the kidney, consists of a glomerular capillary and tubular network, which empties into the collecting duct. There are approximately 1.2 million nephrons per kidney. At rest, only one-tenth of these are required to maintain home-ostasis. The nephrons enable the kidneys to regulate body water and ionic composition, and to excrete waste products and foreign chemicals (e.g. drugs). The nephrons also secrete hormones that participate in the regulation of systemic and renal haemodynamics (renin, angiotensin II, and prostaglandins), haemato-poiesis (erythropoietin), and bone metabolism (calcitriol). Moreover, in the fasting state, they are capable of producing glucose (gluconeogenesis) and participate in the catabolism of peptide hormones.

RENAL BLOOD SUPPLY

The kidneys receive 20–25% of the cardiac output while constituting approximately 0.5% of the total body weight. In terms of flow per 100 g weight, the renal blood flow (RBF) is four times greater than that of the liver or exercising muscle and eight times that of coronary blood flow. The renal cortex (the outer part of the kidney, containing most of the nephrons) receives approximately 75% of the RBF; the rest goes to the medulla. The medulla is the inner part of the kidney and contains specialised nephrons in the juxtamedullary region, immediately next to the medulla. These juxtamedullary nephrons, which have long loops of Henle, are responsible for concentrating the urine when the body needs to conserve water.

Blood enters the kidneys through the renal arteries, which arise from the upper abdominal aorta and passes through serial branches (interlobar, arcuate, and interlobular) before entering the glomeruli via the afferent arterioles. The glomerulus consists of a tuft of capillaries interposed between the afferent and efferent arterioles. Each glomerulus is enclosed within an epithelial cell capsule (Bowman's capsule) that is continuous both with the epithelial cells that surround the glomerular capillaries and with the cells of the proximal convoluted tubule. The glomerular capillaries merge to form the efferent arteriole, which leads to a capillary network that supplies blood to the nephron. The vessels of the venous system run parallel to the arterial vessels and form progressively the interlobular, the arcuate, the interlobar, and the renal veins.

GLOMERULAR FILTRATION

The first step in urine formation begins with the process of glomerular filtration (~180 l/day), which is the ultrafiltration of plasma water (devoid of cellular elements and proteins) from the glomerular capillaries into Bowman's capsule. About 20% of the renal plasma flow is filtered each minute (125 ml/min). This is the glomerular filtration rate (GFR). The composition of the glomerular filtrate (or ultrafiltrate) is identical to plasma with respect to small molecules such as amino acids, glucose, and electrolytes. The filtration barrier prevents the passage of large molecules and cells from the blood in the glomerular capillaries into Bowman's capsule (see below). The driving hydrostatic pressure is controlled by the afferent and efferent arterioles.

Determinants of the GFR

Glomerular ultrafiltration occurs because hydrostatic (P) and osmotic (π) pressures (so-called Starling's forces) drive fluid from the lumen of the glomerular capillaries, across the filtration barrier, into Bowman's capsule. The GFR is determined by the net filtration pressure P_u (the sum of the hydrostatic and colloid osmotic forces across the glomerular membrane), and the glomerular capillary ultrafiltration coefficient K_f:

$$GFR = K_f\, P_u$$

The net ultrafiltration pressure represents the sum of the hydrostatic and colloid osmotic forces that either favour or oppose filtration across the glomerular capillaries.

$$P_u = (P_G - P_B) - (\pi_G - \pi_B)$$

The GFR can therefore be expressed as:

$$GFR = K_f\,[(P_G - P_B) - (\pi_G - \pi_B)]$$

where P_G is the glomerular hydrostatic pressure, P_B is the hydrostatic pressure in Bowman's capsule, outside the capillaries, π_G is the colloid osmotic pressure of the glomerular capillary plasma proteins, and π_B is the colloid osmotic pressure of the proteins in Bowman's capsule.

Because, under normal conditions, the concentration of proteins in the glomerular filtrate is low, the colloid osmotic pressure of the fluid in Bowman's capsule is considered to be zero. Therefore P_G is the only force that favours filtration. Filtration is opposed by the hydrostatic pressure in Bowman's capsule (P_B) and the oncotic pressure in the glomerular capillary (π_G).

The ultrafiltration coefficient K_f is the product of the intrinsic water permeability of the glomerular capillary and the available glomerular surface area. Under normal conditions, GFR can be altered by changing either K_f or any of the Starling forces. Normally the GFR is regulated by alterations in P_G, mediated primarily by changes in glomerular arteriolar resistance. Although increasing K_f raises the GFR, and decreasing it reduces the GFR, changes in K_f are probably not a primary mechanism for the regulation of GFR under normal circumstances. During pathological conditions, however, changes in K_f (especially through loss of filtration surface area) have a profound effect on the GFR.

Filtration barrier

The filtration barrier is composed of three layers:

- the glomerular capillary endothelium;
- the glomerular basement membrane (GBM);
- the epithelium (epithelial cells of Bowman's capsule).

The endothelium has fenestrae or 'pores' with diameters of 70–100 nm, making it relatively permeable even to large molecules. These pores, however, are impermeable to blood cells. The GBM is the primary barrier to the filtration of larger molecules and is the actual filtration barrier, and it excludes most plasma proteins. The capsular epithelial cells (podocytes) are attached to the basement membrane by foot processes, which are separated by filtration slits covered by thin diaphragms. Thus the epithelium may serve as an additional filtration barrier. All components of the filtration barrier are coated with negatively charged glycoproteins, presenting a charge-selective barrier. Besides this charge-selectivity, the filtration barrier is size-selective for large molecules.

AUTOREGULATION AND TUBULOGLOMERULAR FEEDBACK

The GFR and RBF are kept at a relatively constant level by two intrarenal processes: autoregulation and tubuloglomerular feedback.

Autoregulation

The autoregulation of GFR and RBF occurs mainly through variations in afferent arteriolar resistance and changes in distal tubular flow rate. Autoregulation occurs over a wide range of arterial perfusion pressures (80–180 mmHg; Figure 8.1). The mechanism by which the autoregulation is mediated is not completely understood. It is probably an interaction between myogenic responses (through myogenic stretch receptors in the wall of the afferent arteriole), effects of angiotensin II, and tubuloglomerular feedback. In response to changes in arterial pressure, parallel regulation of GFR and RBF results. As systemic pressure rises, an increase in afferent arteriolar tone prevents transmission of the high pressure to the glomerulus. Conversely, as blood pressures

decreases, afferent arteriolar vasodilatation will initially protect both GFR and RBF. However, the GFR and RBF will decrease whenever the mean arterial pressure (MAP) falls below 70 mmHg, and GFR ceases at a MAP of 40–50 mmHg.

Tubuloglomerular feedback

Tubuloglomerular feedback (TGF) refers to alterations in GFR induced by changes in distal tubular flow rate. This mechanism is a function of the juxtaglomerular apparatus (composed of the macula densa cells, smooth muscle cells, and juxtaglomerular cells). The macula densa contains special distal tubular epithelial cells that sense changes in the delivery of chloride. Increased macula densa flow induces the production of renin. Renin converts angiotensinogen (an α_2-globulin produced in the liver) to angiotensin I. Angiotensin I is then converted to angiotensin II by angiotensin-converting enzyme (ACE), present in the lungs, the glomerulus, and vascular endothelial cells. Angiotensin II-mediated afferent arteriolar constriction returns the GFR and macula densa flow towards normal.

The tubule

The tubule has four distinct segments: the proximal tubule, the loop of Henle, the distal tubule, and the connecting duct (Figure 8.2). The proxi-

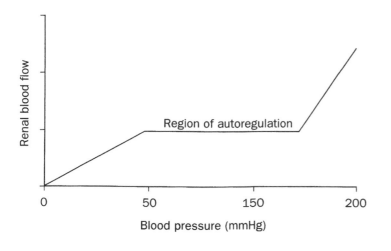

Figure 8.1 Relationship between renal perfusion pressure and renal blood flow. Autoregulation maintains renal blood flow constant as perfusion pressure varies between approximately 50 and 180 mmHg.

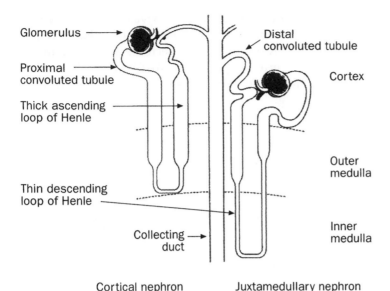

Figure 8.2 *Schematic structure of the renal nephron.*

mal tubule reabsorbs about 60% of the glomerular filtrate, in particular water, electrolytes, bicarbonate, glucose, urea, phosphate, and any filtered proteins. Hydrogen and ammonium ions, urate, and organic anions and cations are secreted from the blood into the proximal tubule. The loop of Henle is divided into descending and ascending limbs. The proximal parts of both limbs have thick walls, like other parts of the nephron, separated by a thin-walled segment. The characteristics of the loops of Henle differ depending on whether they belong to cortical or juxtamedullary nephrons. Cortical nephrons have short loops that penetrate only into the outer zone of the renal medulla, and short terminal thin segments. The loops of juxtamedullary nephrons are much longer, with long thin segments that descend deep into the medulla. The loops of Henle merge with the distal convoluted tubules in the renal cortex. The function of the loop of Henle is to produce a concentrated urine by creating an increasing osmotic gradient in the medulla. This gradient permits reabsorption of water from the collecting ducts. The distal tubules do not reabsorb water, but do reabsorb sodium, chloride, calcium, and bicarbonate ions, and secrete potassium and hydrogen ions into their lumens. Each distal tubule drains into a collecting duct.

Tubular reabsorption and secretion

Approximately 180 l of protein-free glomerular ultrafiltrate is produced each day, 99% of which is reabsorbed (especially water and sodium). As the filtrate passes through the tubules, substances may be removed (reabsorption) or added (secretion). Many of the filtered substances are completely reabsorbed, but some, such as glucose, have a maximum rate of tubular reabsorption (tubular maximum). Many important endogenous and exogenous solutes are secreted into the tubular lumen from the capillary blood. Reabsorption of solutes is by passive transport (diffusion), active mechanisms, or endocytosis. Active transport requires energy to move solutes against an electrochemical or a concentration gradient. It is the main determinant of oxygen consumption by the kidney. As already mentioned, the kidney receives 20% of the total cardiac output but extracts relatively little oxygen. There is, however, a marked discrepancy between the renal cortex and medulla with respect to blood flow, oxygen delivery, and oxygen consumption. The medulla receives only 6% of the RBF and has an average oxygen tension of 1–1.5 kPa. The metabolically active thick ascending loop of Henle in the medulla is therefore particularly vulnerable to hypoxia.

Passive transport

In passive transport, reabsorption occurs down an electrochemical, pressure, or concentration gradient. It develops spontaneously and does not requires energy. Uncharged solutes move from an area of higher concentration to an area of lower concentration (i.e. down their chemical concentration gradient). Additionally, because ions are charged, the passive transport of ions is affected by the electrical potential difference (electrical gradient) across cell membranes and renal tubules. Lipid-soluble substances (e.g. O_2, CO_2, and NH_3) diffuse across the lipid bilayer of the plasma membrane. Diffusion of water (osmosis) occurs through channels in the cell membrane and through so-called tight junctions, and is driven by the osmotic pressure gradient. As water moves across the tight junctions by osmosis, it can also carry some solutes, a process referred to as solvent drag.

Active transport

In active transport, solutes move from an area of lower concentration to an area of higher concentration, and it is coupled directly to energy derived from metabolic processes. The energy for this active transport comes from the hydrolysis of ATP by membrane-bound ATPase. The most prevalent active transport mechanism is the Na^+/K^+-ATPase (or sodium pump), located at the basolateral membrane. Other active transport mechanisms are H^+-ATPase, H^+/K^+-ATPase, and Ca^{2+}-ATPase. H^+-ATPase and H^+/K^+-ATPase are responsible for H^+ secretion in the collecting ducts. Ca^{2+}-ATPase is responsible for the movement of Ca^{2+} from the cytoplasm into the blood. Most solute reabsorption is active, with water being freely permeable and therefore moving by osmosis. When active reabsorption of solute from the tubule occurs, there is a fall in concentration and hence osmotic activity within the tubule. Water then moves, because of osmotic forces, out of the tubule, where the concentration of solutes is higher.

Endocytosis

Endocytosis is another form of active transport. It is the movement of a substance across the cell membrane by a process involving invagination of part of the membrane. It is an important mechanism for reabsorbing small proteins and macromolecules by the proximal tubule.

The proximal tubule

Approximately 60% of the filtered water and most of the solutes (especially Na^+, K^+, and Cl^-) are reabsorbed by the proximal tubule. This includes about 100% of the filtered glucose, HCO_3^- and amino acids as well as some phosphate. In the first part of the proximal tubule, the reabsorption of Na^+ is coupled to that of HCO_3^- and of organic molecules (e.g. glucose and amino acids). In the second part of the tubule, Na^+ reabsorption is coupled to reabsorption of Cl^-. Absorption of Na^+ with organic anions and HCO_3^- in the first part of the proximal tubule results in a relatively high Cl^- concentration, promoting passive entry of Cl^-. The proximal tubule is also an important site of secretion of many endogenous anions (e.g. bile salts and urate), cations (e.g. creatinine and dopamine), and drugs (e.g. diuretics, penicillin, and cimetidine).

The loop of Henle

The loop of Henle is the part of the tubule that loops from the cortex into the medulla (descending limb) before returning to the cortex (ascending limb). The thick ascending loop of Henle reabsorbs about 20% of filtered Na^+, Ka^+, and HCO_3^-. However, the reabsorption of water (approximately 15% of the filtered water) occurs in the descending limb of the loop of Henle. The loop of Henle is the part of the tubule where the urine is concentrated. This is possible because of the high concentration of solutes maintained by the countercurrent multiplier.

The countercurrent mechanism depends on the special anatomical arrangement of the loop of Henle and the vasa recta, the peritubular capillaries of the renal medulla. The countercurrent mechanism occurs primarily in the 25–30% of the nephrons with loops of Henle and vasa recta that penetrate deep into the medulla (the juxtaglomerular nephrons).

The countercurrent multiplier

The excretion of excess solutes by the kidneys, and the production of a concentrated urine, rely on the progressively higher osmotic pressure in the urine and the interstitial fluids as one descends from the renal cortex to the medulla (Figure 8.3). The glomerular filtrate has an osmolality of 300 mosmol/kg, and this increases to 1200–1400 mosmol/kg at the tips of the medullary papillae. The main mechanisms contributing to this osmotic gradient are active transport of Na^+ and other ions into the interstitium by the thick parts of the ascending limb of the loop of Henle and the collecting ducts, and passive diffusion of large amounts of urea from the collecting ducts into the interstitium. The gradient is maintained by the juxtaglomerular nephrons, with their long loops of Henle, which act as a countercurrent multiplier, and by an associated countercurrent exchange mechanism of the vasa recta. The vasa recta, the blood vessels of the loop of Henle, and the collecting ducts, are arranged in a descending and ascending loop tightly applied to the loop of Henle.

An essential factor in the development of the countercurrent mechanism is the difference in permeability and solutes transport of the descending and ascending parts of the loop of Henle. The descending part of the loop of Henle is relatively impermeable to solutes but permeable to water. The thin and thick sections of the ascending loop of Henle are impermeable to water, but permeable to solutes (especially Na^+ and Cl^-). Water moves out of the descending loop by osmosis, increasing the concentration of sodium ions. As the tubule descends, much of this sodium diffuses into the interstitium, further increasing its osmolality. The remaining

sodium is carried back up the ascending limb, which has a very low permeability to water. Here the sodium is actively reabsorbed into the interstitium, while water remains in the tubule, lowering the osmolality of the tubular fluid. This repetitive reabsorption of Na^+ ions, which is added to the continual inflow of newly arriving sodium from the proximal tubule, multiplies the sodium concentration in the lower medulla – hence the name *countercurrent* multiplier.

One might expect that the high solute concentrations in the medulla would be carried away by the blood. Two factors are important in minimising loss of solute. One is the low medullary blood flow, only 1–2% of the total RBF. Secondly, the vasa recta act as countercurrent fluid exchangers. The vasa recta vessels form two parallel arms in close proximity to each other, and are highly permeable to water and solutes, both essential elements in a countercurrent fluid exchange mechanism. Solutes such as sodium and urea diffuse out of interstitium into the blood as the vessels descend into the medulla, while water diffuses in the opposite direction. This results in a progressive increase in the osmolality of the blood as it descends (Figure 8.3). Then, as the blood flows back towards the cortex, almost all the sodium and urea diffuse back into the blood, and water returns to the interstitial fluids. By the time the blood reaches the cortex, it has an osmolar concentration only slightly higher than when it entered the vasa recta, and only minimal amounts of solute are lost. This vascular countercurrent fluid exchange serves to trap solutes in the medullary tissues.

The distal tubule and collecting duct

The distal nephron consists of four segments: the distal tubule, the connecting segment, the cortical collecting tubule, and the medullary collecting tubule. These segments perform different functions and can be separated both by histological appearance and by hormone responsiveness (see below). The distal nephron, particularly the collecting ducts, is the site where the final qualitative changes are made. Thus the maximal

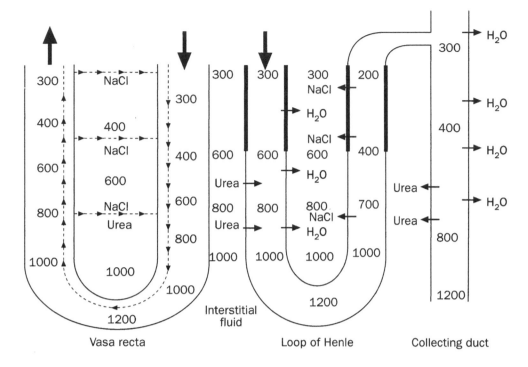

Figure 8.3 *The countercurrent multiplier mechanism responsible for the production of a concentrated urine by the kidneys.*

concentration of the urine, potassium secretion, the maximal acidification of the urine, and sodium concentration all occur in the collecting tubules.

The proximal segment of the distal tubule

This is structurally and functionally similar to the thick ascending loop of Henle. Approximately 5% of the filtered NaCl is reabsorbed at the distal tubule and collecting duct. Water reabsorption depends on the plasma concentration of ADH. Na^+ entry into the cell is primarily mediated by an Na^+/Cl^- cotransporter in the luminal membrane and, to a lesser degree, by a parallel Na^+/H^+ and $Cl^--HCO_3^-$ exchange. The energy for this process is, as elsewhere in the nephron, indirectly provided by the basolateral Na^+/K^+-ATPase pump. NaCl reabsorption can be inhibited by thiazide-type diuretics, through inhibition of the Na^+/Cl^- cotransporter. As with the loop of Henle, distal tubular Na^+ reabsorption varies directly with Na^+ delivery and therefore participates in glomerulotubular balance.

Thus an increase in delivery results in a proportionate rise in Na^+ reabsorption. This effect is independent of hormones such as aldosterone and is, as in the loop of Henle, probably related to changes in the Na^+ concentration in the tubular fluid. Elevation in the luminal Na^+ concentration favours passive Na^+ entry into the tubular cell.

The connecting segment

This lies between the distal tubule and the initial part of the cortical collecting tubule and shares characteristics of both segments. Like the distal tubule, it is impermeable to water, even in the presence of ADH. It reabsorbs Na^+ by a thiazide-sensitive Na^+/Cl^- cotransporter. It also reabsorbs Ca^{2+}, under the influence of both parathyroid hormone (PTH) and calcitriol. Like the cortical collecting tubule, it reabsorbs Na^+ and secretes K^+ in response to aldosterone.

The cortical collecting tubule

This has two cell types with different functions:

the principal cells (about 65%) and the intercalated cells. The principal cells reabsorb Na^+ and water, and secrete K^+, through Na^+ and K^+ channels in the luminal membrane and Na^+/K^+-ATPase pumps in the basolateral membrane. The intercalated cells do not transport NaCl, since they have a lower level of Na^+/K^+-ATPase activity and they have few apical membrane Na^+ channels. They are primarily involved in the regulation of acid–base balance, and either secrete H^+ (reabsorb HCO_3^-) or secrete HCO_3^-. The principal cells can secrete H^+ against a large concentration gradient. Moreover, they play a role in K^+ reabsorption in states of K^+ depletion.

The medullary collecting tubule

This plays an important role in determining the final urine composition of water and solutes. In the first part of this segment, cells such as the principal cells contribute to Na^+ reabsorption and K^+ secretion. The second part is involved in active H^+ secretion via an aldosterone-sensitive H^+-ATPase in the luminal membrane. The water permeability of the medullary collecting tubule is increased by ADH, leading to a more concentrated urine.

ACID–BASE BALANCE

Acid–base balance is accomplished through the coordinated functions of the liver, lungs, and kidneys. An acid is defined as a substance that can donate H^+ ions and a base as a substance that can accept H^+ ions. H^+ regulation is essential because the activity of almost all enzymes in the body is influenced by H^+ concentration. The H^+ concentration is kept at a low level compared with other ions (e.g. Na^+, K^+, Cl^- and HCO_3^-). The normal extracellular hydrogen concentration is approximately 40 nmol/l. In comparison, the concentration of Na^+ is about 3.5 million times greater. Normal variations in H^+ concentration are only about 3–5 nmol/l. Because of the low H^+ concentration of the body fluids, the H^+ concentration is expressed as the negative logarithm, or pH:

$$pH = -\log_{10}[H^+]$$

Thus, with a normal H^+ concentration of 40 nmol/l (0.00000004 mol/l), the pH is

$$pH = -\log[0.00000004] = 7.4$$

It is important to realise that the pH varies inversely with the concentration of H^+. Thus an increase in the H^+ concentration reduces the pH, and a decrease in the concentration elevates the pH. The intracellular pH is usually slightly lower than the plasma pH because metabolism in cells produces acid, especially H_2CO_3. The intracellular pH range is 6.0–7.4. The urine pH varies between 4.5 and 8.0, depending on the acid–base status of the extracellular fluid.

Regulation of the H^+ ion involves three basic steps:

1. Chemical buffering by the extracellular and intracellular buffers, which immediately combine with acid or base to prevent major changes in the H^+ concentration.
2. Control of the partial pressure of carbon dioxide in the body by alterations in alveolar ventilation.
3. Excretion of either acid or bicarbonate through the kidneys.

The buffer system reacts within seconds to minimise changes in pH. The respiratory system reacts within minutes to eliminate CO_2, and therefore H_2CO_3, from the body. The kidneys will eventually eliminate the excess of base or acid from the body. They are, however, slow in their response, reacting over a period of hours to days.

Buffering of hydrogen ions

A buffer is a substance that can reversibly bind H^+. All buffers depend on a simple equilibrium determined by the dissociation constant (K_d or pK_a) of the buffer. The pK_a is the pH at which half of the substance is in ionized form and half un-ionised. The general form of the buffering reaction is

$$buffer + H^+ \leftrightarrow H\text{–}buffer$$

When the H^+ concentration rises, the reaction is forced to the right and more H^+ binds to the buffer. Conversely, when the H^+ concentration decreases, the reaction is forced to the left and H^+ ions are released from the buffer. Several intracellular and extracellular buffer systems exist, of which the bicarbonate system is the most important.

The bicarbonate buffer system

The bicarbonate buffer system differs from the other buffer systems of the body because it is regulated by both the lungs and the kidneys. It can be described by the following reaction:

$$CO_2 + H_2O \overset{CA}{\leftrightarrow} H_2CO_3 \leftrightarrow H^+ + HCO_3^-$$

The first component of the system (hydration/dehydration of CO_2) is the rate-limiting step. The enzyme carbonic anhydrase (CA), present in the wall of the lung alveoli and the proximal renal tubules, greatly accelerates the reaction. The equilibrium of the reaction lies far to the left; there are approximately 340 molecules of CO_2 for each molecule of H_2CO_3. The second component, the ionisation of H_2CO_3 to $H^+ + HCO_3^-$ is virtually instantaneous. Because of the weak dissociation of H_2CO_3, the H^+ concentration is extremely small.

When an acid is added to the extracellular fluid, the H^+ concentration rises, shifting the reaction to the left with the production of more CO_2. This excess CO_2 is eventually eliminated by the respiratory system, thereby enhancing the effectiveness of HCO_3^- buffering. The opposite reaction takes place when a base is added to the buffer solution. CO_2 has a tendency to decrease, but this is counteracted by inhibition of ventilation. The rise in HCO_3^- is compensated for by increased renal excretion of HCO_3^-.

Other buffer systems

Although the bicarbonate buffer system is the principal extracellular buffer, phosphate and plasma proteins provide additional buffering, both extracellular and especially intracellular buffering:

$$H^+ + HPO_4^{2-} \leftrightarrow H_2PO_4^-$$
$$H^+ + protein \leftrightarrow protein^-$$

Because the concentration of phosphate in the extracellular fluid is low, the phosphate buffer system is not an important extracellular buffer, but it does play a major role in the renal tubular fluid and intracellular fluid. The concentration of phosphate in the renal tubules and intracellularly is high. Moreover, the pH is lower than that of the extracellular fluid and therefore closer to the pK_a (6.8) of the phosphate buffer system. The proteins in the body function as bases because they possess negatively charged amino acids that readily accept H^+. Haemoglobin in red blood cells is one of the important body bases. The combined action of the HCO_3^-, phosphate, and plasma protein buffering systems account for approximately 50% of the buffering of the acid load and for 70% of the base load.

Respiratory regulation of acid–base balance

The second line of defence against acid–base disturbances is control of extracellular fluid CO_2 concentration by the lungs. An increase in ventilation eliminates CO_2 from the extracellular fluid, thereby reducing the H^+ concentration. Conversely, decreased ventilation increases CO_2 and H^+ concentration. The H^+ concentration itself also affects the alveolar ventilation. A decrease in pH increases the alveolar ventilation. When the plasma pH rises above 7.4, ventilation is decreased. Because increased H^+ concentration stimulates the alveolar ventilation, and because increased alveolar ventilation in turn decreases the H^+ concentration, the respiratory system acts as a negative-feedback mechanism. However, it is not capable on its own of normalising the H^+ concentration.

Renal regulation of acid–base balance

The kidney contributes to the acid–base balance by excreting an amount of acid equal to the production of non-volatile acids, mainly from the metabolism of proteins. Furthermore, the kidney prevents loss of HCO_3^- in the urine – a task that is quantitatively more important than excretion of non-volatile acids. Both reabsorption of filtered HCO_3^- and excretion of acids are accomplished through tubular H^+ secretion. It is essential to appreciate that loss of filtered HCO_3^- in the urine is equivalent to the addition of H^+ ions to the body, since both are derived from the dissociation of H_2CO_3. As a result, almost all of the filtered HCO_3^- must be reabsorbed before the dietary H^+ load can be excreted. Approximately 4390 mmol/day of H^+ is secreted into the tubular fluid. Most of this is utilised in the process of reabsorbing the filtered HCO_3^-, and about 80 mmol is excreted.

Hydrogen secretion and bicarbonate reabsorption

H^+ secretion and HCO_3^- reabsorption occur in virtually all parts of the tubules except the descending and ascending thin limbs of the loop of Henle. About 80% of HCO_3^- reabsorption occurs in the proximal tubule. An additional 10–15% of the filtered load is reabsorbed at the thick ascending part of the loop of Henle, and the remainder of the reabsorption takes place in the distal tubule and collecting duct. HCO_3^- reabsorption (and secretion) is regulated by several factors, of which the Na^+ balance and aldosterone are the most important. The primary sites of regulation are the proximal tubule and collecting duct.

HORMONAL CONTROL OF TUBULAR REABSORPTION

The regulation of blood pressure, intravascular volume, and salt and water homeostasis are regulated by two interrelated neurohormonal systems. The sympathoadrenal axis, the renin–angiotensin–aldosterone system, and antidiuretic hormone (ADH) promote vasoconstriction and salt and water preservation. Prostaglandins, bradykinins, and atrial natriuretic peptide (ANP), on the other hand, promote vasodilatation and salt and water excretion.

The sympathicoadrenal axis

Sympathetic nerve fibres innervate the afferent and efferent arterioles of the glomerulus. The primary stimulus for the sympathetic response (through circulating adrenaline and neuronal release of noradrenaline) is a decrease in effective circulating volume (ECV). A decrease in ECV (sensed by baroreceptors in the aortic arch, carotid sinus and afferent arteriole) leads to an increase in renal sympathetic activity. This has the following effects: (1) afferent and efferent vasoconstriction leading to a decrease in GFR and therefore a reduction in the filtered load of Na^+, (2) activation of the renin–angiotensin–aldosterone system, and (3) NaCl reabsorption (especially at the proximal tubule) by both a direct adrenergic effect and increases in angiotensin II and aldosterone activity.

The renin–angiotensin–aldosterone system

The juxtaglomerular cells (with distal tubular and macula densa cells, part of the juxtaglomerular apparatus) synthesise the precursor prorenin, which is cleaved into the active proteolytic enzyme renin. The production of renin is stimulated by three important mechanisms: (1) primarily by a decrease in renal artery perfusion pressure, (2) sympathetic nervous stimulation of the afferent arterioles, and (3) delivery of NaCl to the macula densa. An increase in Cl^- concentration in the tubular fluid triggers renin release from the afferent arterioles. This tubuloglomerular feedback mechanism keeps the delivery of solutes (especially NaCl) to the distal tubule at a constant level.

Renin acts on angiotensinogen, a circulating glycloprotein produced by the liver, and cleaves off a decapeptide, angiotensin I. In the lungs and kidneys, angiotensin I is further cleaved to an octapeptide, angiotensin II, by a surface-bound vascular endothelial enzyme (angiotensin-converting enzyme, ACE). Activated angiotensin II causes predominantly afferent arteriole vasoconstriction. This acts to maintain the GFR in the face of mild to moderate decreases in RBF or renal perfusion pressure. Angiotensin II further stimulates secretion of aldosterone and

ADH and reabsorption of NaCl in the proximal tubule. Moreover, angiotensin II triggers a number of mechanisms that modulate its actions. It inhibits renin secretion by a negative-feedback mechanism. It activates the synthesis of intrarenal prostaglandins, which counteracts the action of angiotensin II, by preferential efferent arteriole vasodilatation. Moreover, angiotensin II increases atrial pressure and releases ANP, which opposes the renin–angiotensin–aldosterone system.

Aldosterone is a steroid hormone secreted by the zona glomerulosa of the adrenal cortex in response to hypokalaemia, angiotensin II, and adrenocorticotrophic hormone (ACTH). The primary site of action is on the principal cells of the distal tubule and the collecting tubule. Aldosterone stimulates Na^+-K^+-ATPase at the basolateral side and increases the number of open Na^+ and K^+ channels at the luminal membrane, promoting Na^+ reabsorption and K^+ secretion. Moreover, aldosterone stimulates H^+ secretion by activation of luminal H^+-ATPase (especially of the cortical intercalated cells and medullary tubular cells).

ADH is a nine-amino-acid peptide, 8-arginine-vasopressin, synthesised in the supraoptic and paraventricular nuclei of the anterior hypothalamus and secreted at the posterior lobe of the pituitary. It is the primary determinant of renal water excretion. The major stimuli to ADH secretion are hyperosmolality (especially the plasma Na^+ concentration) and a decrease in the ECV (mediated by stretch receptors in the left atrium and pulmonary veins). Hypovolaemia-induced secretion of ADH overrides osmolar responses. ADH augments the water permeability (through a specific V_2 receptor) of the luminal membranes of the cortical and medullary collecting tubules, allowing osmotic equilibration with the interstitium. It also increases NaCl reabsorption in the thick ascending loop of Henle, which maintains the hypertonicity of the medullary interstitium and facilitates the movement of water of the collecting tubule along the osmotic gradient. The final concentration of urine depends upon the amount of ADH. If ADH is present in the distal tubule, the col-lecting duct becomes permeable to water. As the collecting duct passes through the medulla with a high solute concentration in the interstitium, water moves out of the lumen of the duct and concentrated urine is formed. In the absence of ADH, the tubule is minimally permeable to water, resulting in the formation of large quantities of dilute urine.

ANP is released from granules in atrial myocytes in response to local wall stretch and increased atrial volume. ANP has two major actions: systemic vasodilatation, and natriuresis and diuresis (urinary Na^+ and water excretion). The natriuretic and diuretic effects of this hormone are mediated by both renal and extrarenal changes. ANP directly increases the GFR (probably through both afferent arteriolar dilation and efferent arteriolar constriction) and reduces Na^+ reabsorption; this natriuretic action appears to be primarily due to the inhibition of sodium reabsorption in the medullary collecting tubule. Furthermore, ANP opposes the renin–angiotensin–aldosterone system in several ways. It inhibits renin secretion and decreases angiotensin-stimulated aldosterone release. It also inhibits ADH release from the posterior pituitary and antagonises its effects on the V_2 receptor in the collecting tubule, thus promoting diuresis.

Prostaglandins are derived from the metabolism of arachidonic acid, and play an important role in renal protection. They have both vascular (primary vasodilatation) and tubular (water and Na^+ excretion) actions. They are produced at different sites within the kidney, including glomerular and vascular endothelium, the medullary collecting tubule cells, and medullary interstitial cells. Renal prostaglandins have local functions but little systemic activity, since they are rapidly metabolised in the pulmonary circulation. The important vasodilatory renal prostaglandins are PGD_2, PGE_2, and PGI_2 (prostacyclin). They oppose the actions of noradrenaline and angiotensin II, antagonise the effects of ADH, and block distal tubule sodium reabsorption. Phospholipase A_2 (at the inner lipid layer of the cell membrane) controls the prostaglandin production. Arachidonic acid is converted to PGG_2, the precursor of the vasodilator prostaglandins, by cyclooxygenase (COX), which is inhibited by non-steroidal anti-inflammatory drugs (NSAIDs) such as aspirin and indomethacin. NSAIDs do not impair renal perfusion in normal situations but can lead to (ir)reversible renal insufficiency, particularly in hypovolaemic states in which angiotensin II and noradrenaline are stimulated.

Parathyroid hormone (PTH) is a polypeptide secreted by the parathyroid glands in response to a decrease in the plasma concentration of ionised Ca^{2+}. PTH increases the plasma Ca^{2+} concentration in three ways: (1) it stimulates bone resorption (in the presence of vitamin D), resulting in the release of calcium and phosphate; (2) it enhances intestinal Ca^{2+} and phosphate absorption by promoting the formation within the kidney of calcitriol (1,25-dihydroxycholecalciferol); and (3) it augments active renal Ca^{2+} reabsorption, primarily at the distal tubule and connecting segment. PTH also influences phosphate balance. It tends to increase phosphate entry into the extracellular fluid by its effects on bone and intestinal absorption. However, PTH also reduces proximal tubular phosphate reabsorption, resulting in enhanced excretion. The urinary effect usually predominates in patients with relatively normal renal function, as PTH tends to lower the plasma phosphate concentration.

BLADDER FUNCTION AND MICTURITION

The bladder is a smooth muscle chamber composed of two parts; the fundus, which stores the urine, and the neck, which is a funnel-shaped extension of the fundus, connecting to the urethra (the posterior urethra). Bladder smooth muscle is called the detrusor. Detrusor fibres extend in all directions. At the bladder neck, it forms the internal sphincter. This is not a true sphincter but rather a thickening of the bladder wall formed by converging muscle fibres. The urethra passes through the urogenital diaphragm, which contains a layer of muscle called the external sphincter. This is a voluntary skeletal muscle. Urine eventually leaves the urethra through the external meatus.

Innervation of the bladder

The innervation of the bladder and urethra is important in controlling urination. This occurs through pelvic (parasympathetic), pudendal, and hypogastric (sympathetic) nerves. The smooth muscle of the bladder neck and urethra receives sympathetic innervation from the hypogastric nerves. α-Adrenergic stimulation induces muscle contraction and closure of the urethra, which facilitates storage of urine. Pelvic motor nerve (parasympathetic) fibres innervate the fundus of the bladder and cause bladder contraction. Sensory fibres of the pelvic nerves detect the level of bladder wall stretch and are responsible for the initiation of a reflex that empties the bladder. Pudendal (skeletal motor) nerve fibres innervate the voluntary skeletal muscles of the external sphincter, and cause external sphincter contraction.

Micturition

Micturition is the process by which the urinary bladder empties when it becomes filled. Two processes are involved: progressive filling of the bladder until the pressure rises to a threshold level, and a neuronal reflex called the micturition reflex, which empties the bladder. The micturition reflex is an automatic spinal cord reflex, but it can be inhibited or facilitated by centres in the brainstem and the cerebral cortex.

Bladder filling stretches the bladder wall and triggers the micturition reflex initiated by stretch receptors. Sensory signals from the bladder fundus enter the spinal cord via pelvic nerve fibres. Stimulation of parasympathetic fibres causes contraction of the detrusor muscle and muscles in the neck of the bladder. Because the muscle fibres of the bladder outlet are oriented both longitudinally and radially, contraction opens the bladder neck and allows urine to flow through the posterior urethra. Voluntary relaxation of the external sphincter, through cortical inhibition of the pudendal nerve, permits the flow of urine through the external meatus.

9

Physiology of the liver

Bart van Hoek

INTRODUCTION

The liver is one of the most important organs in the body, performing a variety of physiological functions. In addition to its secretory and excretory functions responsible for the formation of bile, it is the main metabolic powerhouse of the body. More than 500 metabolic functions occur in a single hepatocyte. Regulation of these processes takes place at organ level, cellular level, within organelles, and at molecular level. The gallbladder functions in close harmony with the liver. In this chapter, the most important processes are summarised.

FUNCTIONAL ANATOMY AND BLOOD SUPPLY OF THE LIVER

A normal liver weighs 1.2–1.6 kg in an adult, approximately 2% of body weight, but receives about 30% of resting cardiac output. It has eight distinct segments, each with a separate blood supply and biliary drainage (Figure 9.1). The liver consists mainly of hepatocytes organised in acini and lobules. These cells, together with sinusoidal cells, bile duct cells, Ito cells, Kupffer cells, and other immune cells, contribute to the many hepatic functions. The hepatocytes are in close contact with the blood flowing through sinusoids, covered with endothelial cells, and with the space of Disse between endothelium and hepatocytes (Figure 9.2). Hepatocytes display metabolic heterogeneity according to their zonal location within the acinus. Periportal hepatocytes are mainly involved in metabolic protein synthesis; those in the centrilobar zone contain high concentrations of cytochrome P450 and are important for drug biotransformation. Blood from the splenic and superior mesenteric veins draining the bowel enters the liver by the portal vein. Oxygenated blood is supplied by the hepatic artery. Three liver veins form the outflow tract to the inferior vena cava from all but one lobe, the caudate lobe, which has its own venous drainage. Each acinus has a portal triad containing a branch of the hepatic artery, the portal vein, and a bile duct. Blood from the portal venules drains into the hepatic sinusoids and thence into the central vein (Figure 9.3). Between two hepatocytes lies the bile canaliculus (Figure 9.4), which drains into bile ducts. The left and right hepatic bile ducts form the common hepatic duct, which joins the cystic duct from the gallbladder to form the common bile duct. This conveys bile to the duodenum through the sphincter of Oddi (Figure 9.5).

FUNCTIONS OF THE GALLBLADDER AND THE ROLE OF BILE

Between meals, when the sphincter of Oddi is contracted and the smooth muscular wall of the gallbladder is relaxed, bile is stored and concentrated in the gallbladder. Passage of a meal into the duodenum releases the hormone cholecystokinin (CCK), which contracts the gallbladder and relaxes the sphincter of Oddi, allowing con-

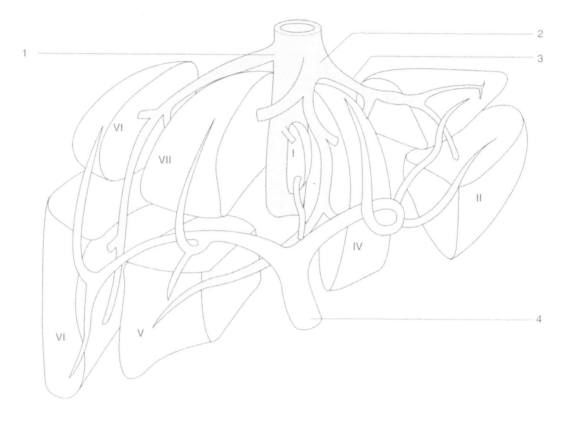

Figure 9.1 *Segmental anatomy of the liver. 1, 2, 3: liver veins; 4: portal vein.*

centrated bile to flow into the duodenum and mix with food. One of the important functions of bile is the formation of micelles, facilitating the absorption of cholesterol, triglycerides, and fat-soluble vitamins and keeping them in 'solution' in the aqueous milieu of the gut, enabling lipase to digest lipids.

FORMATION OF BILE

Approximately 450 ml of canalicular bile is formed daily. To this is added about 150 ml of ductular bile, rich in bicarbonate, resulting in a daily bile production of approximately 600 ml. Ductular bile (so-called 'liver bile') comprises 82% water and 18% solutes, mainly bile acids (bile salts) (67%), phospholipids (22%), protein (5%), cholesterol (4%), and bilirubin (0.3%). Bile

production is lower at night than during the day.

Bile acid production is 400–500 mg/day, mostly excreted in the faeces (Figure 9.6). Excretion in the urine is less than 0.5 mg/day. Bile acids undergo enterohepatic circulation, with reuptake of 95% in the terminal ileum. In the blood, bile acids are bound to albumin or high-density lipoprotein (HDL).

Polypeptides and glycoproteins with strong affinity for bile acids mediate uptake into hepatocytes, an active process against an electrochemical gradient, with energy supply by Na^+–K^+-ATPase. Normally only 1% of the bile acids are present in the peripheral blood, and this does not increase even after meals; an increased concentration only occurs when cholestasis is present.

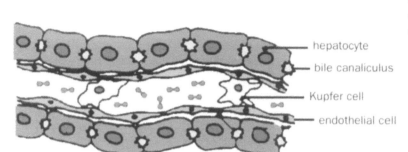

Figure 9.2 *Structure of a liver sinusoid, showing the relationship to a hepatocyte.*

— hepatocyte

— bile canaliculus

— Kupfer cell

— endothelial cell

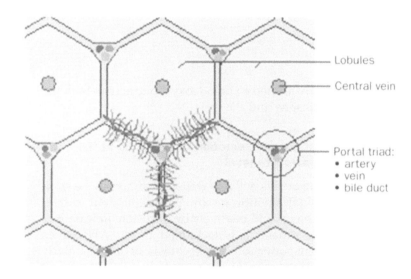

Figure 9.3 *Lobules, central vein, and portal triad.*

— Lobules

— Central vein

— Portal triad:
  • artery
  • vein
  • bile duct

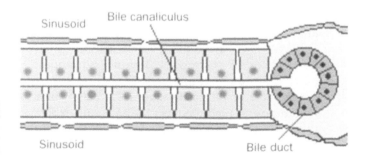

Figure 9.4 *Bile canaliculus and bile duct.*

Sinusoid

Bile canaliculus

Sinusoid

Bile duct

Figure 9.5 *The anatomy of the biliary system.*

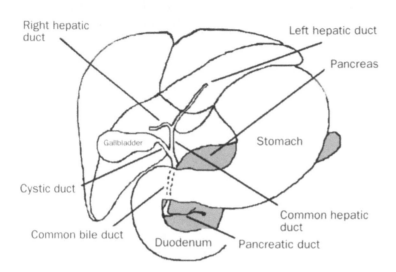

BILE ACID SYNTHESIS

The primary bile acids are formed in the hepatocytes as liver-specific degradation products of cholesterol to cholic acid and chenodeoxycholic acid (Figure 9.7). Twice as much cholic acid as chenodeoxycholic acid is produced, and together they represent 60–90% of total bile production. Bile acids then undergo conjugation with either glycine or taurine to form the water-soluble glycocholic acid, taurocholic acid, glycocheodeoxycholic acid, and taurochenodeoxycholic acid, which together represent 72% of conjugated primary bile acids (Figure 9.8). Bile acids re-entering the liver after passage through the enterohepatic circulation inhibit their own synthesis (negative feedback).

The secondary bile acids (Figure 9.7) result from deconjugation by anaerobic gut flora in the ileum, caecum, and colon with release of free bile acids. These are partially (30–50%) absorbed in the intestine, and following reconjugation in the liver are again excreted into the canaliculi, so that the bile contains a mixture of primary and secondary bile acids.

The tertiary bile acids are formed in both the liver and the gut. Lithocholic acid absorbed from the intestine is converted to sulpholithocholic acid in the liver. Ketolithocholic acid is transformed to ursodeoxycholic acid in both the intestine and the liver.

Uptake and secretion of bile acids at the hepatocyte level

Bile acid is actively transported across the sinusoidal membrane by Na^+-dependent carrier proteins and passively by diffusion. Release into the canaliculi is facilitated by an ATP-driven transporter, or by exocytosis of intracellularly derived mixed vesicles and potential-dependent membrane carriers (Figure 9.6).

NTCP (sodium taurocholate cotransporting protein) is the main uptake carrier for bile salts in the liver. Other proteins involved are organic anion transporting proteins (OATP2 and OATP8). These have other functions, including the uptake of oestrogens, thyroid hormones, bilirubin, and digoxin.

Secretion of bile salts across the canalicular membrane is mediated by the bile salt export pump (BSEP), a protein belonging to the family of ATP-binding cassette transporters (ABC transporters). Other bile components such as phospholipids, cholesterol, conjugated bilirubin, and many drugs and toxins are also transported to the canaliculus by ABC transporters (Figure 9.6).

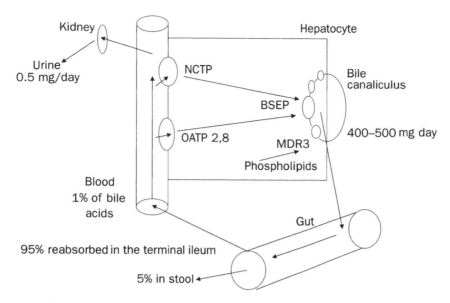

Figure 9.6 *The enterohepatic circulation of bile acids with relevant ABC transporters. BSEP: bile salt export pump; NCTP: sodium taurocholate cotransporting pump; OATP: organic anion transporting proteins. MRP2 transports conjugated bilirubin, ABCG5/G8 transports cholesterol and MDR3 is a flippase for phospholipids.*

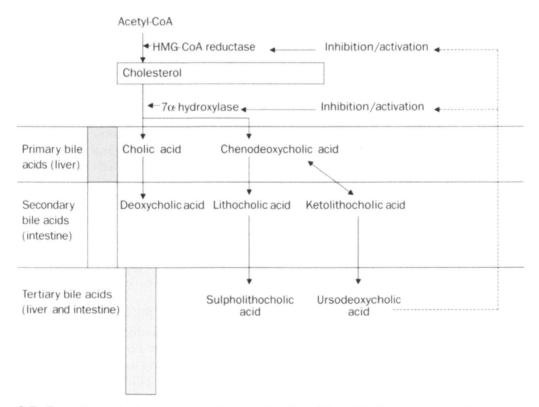

Figure 9.7 *Formation of primary, secondary, and tertiary bile acids from cholesterol.*

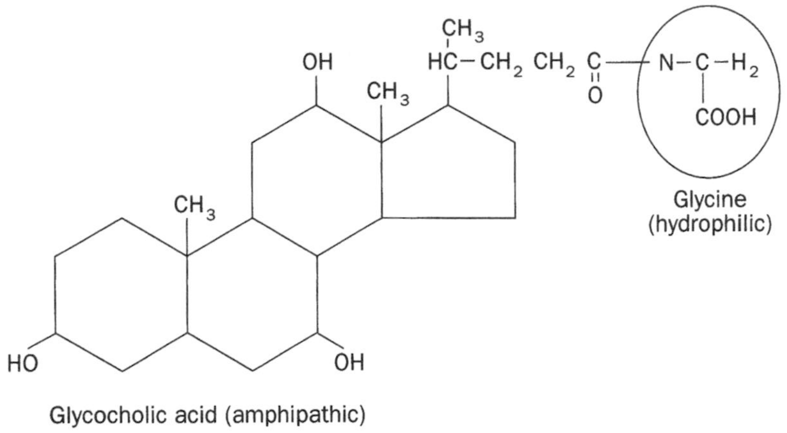

Figure 9.8 *Formation of glycocholic acid from cholic acid.*

Glycine
(hydrophilic)

Glycocholic acid (amphipathic)

PORPHYRIN METABOLISM

Porphyrins are the prosthetic groups of haemo-proteins (haemoglobin, myoglobin, cytochromes, etc.). Haem synthesised in the erythrocyte is a precursor for the synthesis of haemoglobin and, in the hepatocytes, for the synthesis of hepatic haemoproteins, especially cytochrome P450. Daily production of haem amounts to about 300 mg, of which only 1% is excreted unused in the urine and stools. The porphyrinogens are colourless intermediate products of haem synthesis. Oxidation leads to the red-fluorescing porphyrins. Haem synthesis is regulated by three enzymes: δ-aminolaevulinic acid (ALA) synthase, uroporphyrinogen decarboxylase, and ferrochelatase (Figure 9.9). The most crucial enzyme, δ-ALA synthase, is inhibited by haem. Porphyrins are irreversible oxidation products that, with the exception of protoporphyrin, are not utilised for other purposes, but are excreted. Under pathological conditions, they are stored in cells. Some intermediate products are eliminated in the stools (e.g. protoporphyrin IX) and others in the urine (e.g. coproporphyrin III and uroporphyrin I). Important inducers of δ-ALA synthase include barbiturates, sulphonamides, oestrogens, androgens, alcohol, and fasting.

BILIRUBIN METABOLISM

Bilirubin is derived primarily from haem by the breakdown of ageing erythrocytes in the spleen, liver, kidneys, and bone marrow, while 20–30% comes from the degradation of other metallo-porphyrins. It is water-insoluble and potentially toxic. It is bound to serum albumin and transported to the sinusoidal membrane of the liver cell as a bilirubin–albumin complex (Figure 9.10). Albumin binds to the hepatocyte cell membrane, and uncoupling of bilirubin follows. Active bilirubin uptake into the liver cell is mediated by non-specific membrane glycoproteins.

The binding capacity of albumin is exceeded only at serum bilirubin concentrations greater than 4–5 mg/dl. In the case of decreased albumin binding (e.g. in acidosis) or oversaturated binding capacity, toxic cell damage may occur due to the diffusion of unbound bilirubin into cells (accompanied in some cases by kernicterus). Neonates and premature babies are at particular risk because of their immature blood–brain barrier. A precursory bilirubin is formed during the first 3 days of life from the breakdown of erythrocyte precursors in the bone marrow. A smaller proportion originates from haemoproteins in the liver. With increased erythropoiesis or in dyserythropoiesis, the proportion of precursory or indirect bilirubin is raised.

In the hepatocyte, bilirubin is bound to Y protein (identical to glutathione-S-transferase). This prevents its movement from the cytosol into the cellular organelles and its diffusion back into the blood. With a higher bilirubin concentration and saturation of Y protein, bilirubin is also bound to Z protein (fatty acid-binding protein). Within

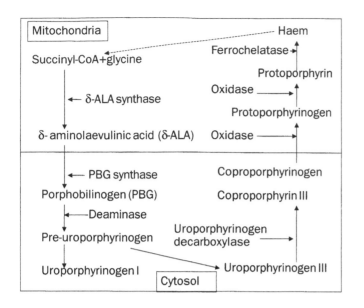

Figure 9.9 Porphyrin metabolism. Modified after Kuntz E, Kuntz HD. Clinical Hepatol 2001, with permission.

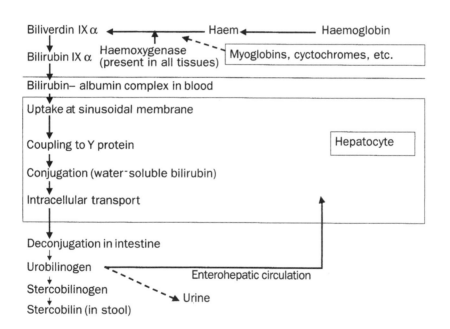

Figure 9.10 Bilirubin metabolism.

the hepatocyte, bilirubin is conjugated with glucuronic acid. Conjugation converts *water-insoluble* primary bilirubin to *water-soluble* secondary bilirubin, which is eliminated via the bile and urine. The conjugated form of bilirubin is normally present in the blood as 3–10% of the total serum bilirubin. Active excretion occurs at the canalicular membrane, whereby bilirubin is concentrated approximately 100-fold. Absorption is possible neither from the gallbladder nor from the intestine, and no enterohepatic reabsorption of bilirubin takes place.

Glucuronic acid is released by β-glucuronidase from enteric bacteria. Bilirubin is converted into colourless urobilinogen by bacterial reductases. Oxidation of urobilinogen gives rise to urobilin and stercobilin, which, together with their degradation products, are responsible for the brown colour of stools. A portion of the urobilinogen is reabsorbed, transported through the portal vein back to the liver, and re-excreted via the bile. A small proportion of the urobilinogen in the blood is eliminated in the urine.

Carbohydrate metabolism

The liver contributes in four different ways to the maintenance of glucose homeostasis: glycogenesis (process of glycogen formation), glycogenolysis (glycogen breakdown to glucose), gluconeogenesis (formation of carbohydrates from proteins and fats), and glucolysis.

After a meal, the liver takes up glucose and uses it for glycolysis or the formation of glycogen. The liver releases glucose from the breakdown of glycogen and from gluconeogenesis for utilisation by peripheral tissues, mainly the brain and erythrocytes, but also by muscle cells, and for storage in adipocytes. Glucose, fructose, and galactose are the basic carbohydrates. Fructose and galactose are converted to glucose in the liver and channelled into glycogenesis. The metabolisation of fructose is insulin-dependent, whereas that of galactose is insulin-independent. Glucose is converted to glucose-6-phosphate and glucose-1-phosphate. From these, UDP-glucose is synthesised, from which glycogen is formed. During hypoglycaemia, a protein phosphorylase is activated by glucagon and adrenaline via cyclic adenosine monophosphate (cAMP). As a result, glycogenesis is inhibited and glycogenolysis is stimulated: glycogen is converted to glucose-1-phosphate, which is then converted to glucose-6-phosphate, and finally free glucose is released.

After ingestion of a meal, the liver retains at least 50% of an oral glucose load for glycogen synthesis and other metabolic functions. Glucose is not taken up directly by the liver but is first released into the circulation by an indirect pathway and taken up by peripheral tissues, where glycolysis to gluconeogenic precursors (e.g. lactate and pyruvate) takes place. These precursors are then released into the circulation, taken up by the liver, and converted to glucose via gluconeogenesis. The glucose is then incorporated into glycogen.

Glucose uptake by hepatocytes is by facilitated diffusion via hepatic glucose transporters – a process that is independent of insulin. Glucose is then converted to glucose-6-phosphate by glucokinase (Figure 9.11). Under physiological conditions, this enzyme is not saturated, so that the capacity of the liver to maintain sinusoidal glucose concentration is independent of hormonal control. The rate-limiting enzymes in hepatic glycogen synthesis and breakdown are glycogen synthase and glycogen phosphorylase (Figure 9.12). High sinusoidal glucose levels lead to inactivation of phosphorylase, which in turn activates glycogen synthase, so that glycogen is synthesised. This occurs within two minutes of an increase in glucose concentration. Glucose may also directly activate glycogen synthase. Although insulin influences the synthesis of glycogen, the intrahepatic glucose concentration is more important in regulating glycogen metabolism after meals.

The liver glycogen storage (around 70 g for an adult) is only enough to meet the 24-hour glucose requirement of the brain (145 g) and other glycolytic tissue (35 g) for 10 hours or, in conjunction with gluconeogenesis, for up to 20 hours. During periods of fasting, the glycogen content falls to 0.1%, but rises to over 10% when a high-carbohydrate diet is consumed. Some 120–150 g of glycogen are stored in the muscles, but this is solely for utilisation by the muscle tissue. With brief fasting (<24 hours), the degradation of hepatic glycogen accounts for 50–75% of hepatic glucose output, and gluconeogenesis for the remainder. As the fast continues and hepatic glycogen is depleted, gluconeogenesis accounts for up to 98% of hepatic glucose output at 2 days.

The three alternative substrates available for glucose synthesis are lactate (60%) from anaerobic glycolysis, amino acids, principally alanine (30%), from proteolysis, and glycerol (10%) from

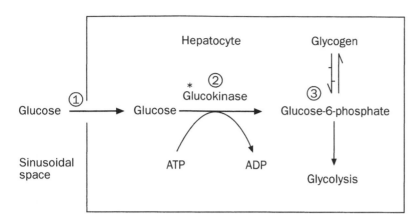

Figure 9.11 *Glucose uptake by the hepatocyte and formation of glucose-6-phosphate as an intermediate in glycogen formation and breakdown and glycolysis. (Derived from Katbamna BH et al. in Zakim D, Boyer TD (eds). Hepatology. A textbook of liver disease. 2nd edn. Philadelphia: WB Saunders, 1990: 73–84. Reprinted with permission.)*

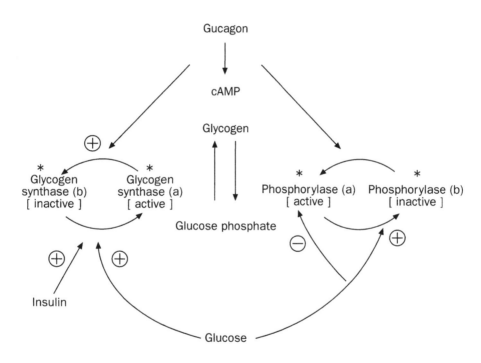

Figure 9.12 *The rate-limiting enzymes in hepatic glycogen synthesis and breakdown are glycogen synthase and glycogen phosphorylase. High sinusoidal glucose levels lead to inactivation of phosphorylase, which in turn activates glycogen synthase, so that glycogen is synthesised. (Derived from Katbamna BH et al. in Zakim D, Boyer TD (eds). Hepatology. A textbook of liver disease. 2nd edn. Philadelphia: WB Saunders, 1990: 73–84. Reprinted with permission.)*

lipolysis in fatty tissue. A short-term rise in gluconeogenesis is stimulated by a fall of the plasma insulin level to 25% of the postprandial level during fasting. Apart from insulin, gluconeogenesis is also controlled by glucagon, which stimulates phosphoenolpyruvate carboxykinase (PEPCK), the rate-limiting enzyme of gluconeogenesis (Figure 9.13). A long-term increase in gluconeogenesis is induced by glucocorticoids, whereas insulin inhibits gluconeogenesis. The key enzymes of glycolysis are activated by insulin, converting catabolic to anabolic metabolism. Ketogenesis in the liver is the result of an increased lipolysis in fatty tissue, with a rise in fatty acids, which occurs during fasting. A portion is converted to ketones for utilisation by the brain and other tissues, but most are passively cleared by the liver. Insulin inhibits ketogenesis.

LIPID AND LIPOPROTEIN METABOLISM

Fats and fat-like compounds may be divided into simple lipids (triglycerides, free fatty acids, free cholesterol, cholesterol esters, and bile acids) and complex lipids (glycerophospholipids and sphingolipids). The medium-chain fatty acids (C6–C12) are transported by the portal vein directly to the liver. Chylomicrons, formed from exogenously derived triglycerides and long-chain fatty acids (C16–C20) in the intestinal mucosa, transport exogenous triglycerides in the lymph and blood. Their contents are released to the tissues by the action of triglyceride lipase and lipoprotein lipase. Chylomicrons are taken up by the liver as cholesterol-rich 'remnants' and degraded in lysosomes. Lipoproteins formed in the liver and in the mucosa of the small intestine transport water-insoluble lipids in the blood, with the exception of the albumin-bound free fatty acids.

Very low-density lipoproteins (VLDL) are mainly synthesised in the liver cell and transport triglycerides of endogenous origin. Low-density lipoproteins (LDL_2) are β lipoproteins formed from VLDL in the plasma (by the action of lipoprotein lipase) via intermediate-density lipoproteins (LDL_1 or IDL). LDL transport cholesterol and cholesterol esters. Hepatocyte LDL receptors take up LDL-bound cholesterol (50–60%) according to cellular requirements. When there is increased LDL availability, macrophages can also clear cholesterol. High-density lipoproteins (HDL) are formed in the liver and small intestine and transport cholesterol esters derived from the action of lecithin-cholesterol-acetyl transferase (LCAT).

Oxidative energy in the liver is generated by β oxidation of short-chain fatty acids and amino acids in the mitochondria via the citrate cycle, and also by the oxidation of fructose and ethanol. The peroxisomes, also involved in β oxidation, produce acetyl-CoA, which is subsequently oxidised to CO_2 in the citrate cycle.

Lipogenesis, the synthesis of lipids from carbohydrate via acetyl-CoA, occurs almost exclusively in the liver cells and fatty tissue. The level of hepatic synthesis is regulated primarily by the insulin–glucagon quotient. Thirteen different apolipoproteins are necessary for lipid metabolism, with great variety in biochemistry and function. Free fatty acids, potentially toxic to the liver cell, are immobilised by being bound to hepatic fatty acid-binding protein (hFABP) in the cytosol.

The liver synthesises triglycerides, which are released as VLDL bodies. There is normally no storage in the hepatocytes. VLDL triglycerides are transported to the white fatty tissue, where they are enzymatically split to allow storage of the resulting fatty acids as triglycerides in the adipocytes. Degradation of triglycerides stored in the fatty tissue is effected by means of lipase and hormonal actions (catecholamines, ACTH, and glucagon).

Free fatty acids influence the rate of VLDL synthesis and hence the triglyceride concentration. About 16 g of glycerol, which is principally utilised in the liver, is released daily by lipolysis, and about 120 g of free fatty acids are made available for generation of energy in the heart and skeletal muscles as well as in the liver. These saturated and unsaturated free fatty acids are bound in the plasma to albumin and lipoproteins. Their plasma half-life is only 2 minutes.

Cholesterol is an important substance for the structure and function of biomembranes. It is also the initial substrate for the biosynthesis of bile acids, vitamin D_3 and steroid hormones. The body synthesises 3.2 mmol/day cholesterol, of which 97% is formed in the liver (85%) and intestine (12%). The cholesterol pool (in liver, plasma, and erythrocytes) is 5.2 mmol/day. Cholesterol is removed from the pool by release into the bile or, as VLDL and HDL particles, into the plasma. The key enzyme in cholesterol synthesis is hydroxymethylglutaryl-CoA reductase (HGM-CoA reductase). Cholesterol esters are formed in the plasma by linking of a lecithin

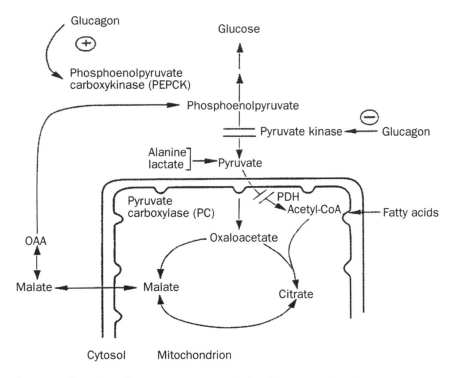

Figure 9.13 *Apart from insulin, gluconeogenesis is also controlled by glucagon, which stimulates phosphoenolpyruvate carboxykinase (PEPCK), the rate-limiting enzyme of gluconeogenesis. (Derived from Katbamna BH et al. in Zakim D, Boyer TD (eds).* Hepatology. A textbook of liver disease. *2nd edn. Philadelphia: WB Saunders, 1990: 73–84. Reprinted with permission.)*

fatty acid to free cholesterol. Endogenous consumption, degradation, and elimination of cholesterol are kept in balance with dietary intake, endogenous synthesis, and intestinal reabsorption.

AMINO ACID AND PROTEIN METABOLISM

The body contains approximately 14 kg of protein. There is a 24-hour turnover of 600–700 g of the amino acid pool. Muscles have the highest absolute rate of protein synthesis (for local use) but, in relation to its weight, the liver generates more protein than muscles (120 g/day). Plasma protein turnover is 25 g/day and total tissue protein turnover 150 g/day. Of the 20 important amino acids, eight are essential, i.e. the body cannot synthesise them, so they must either be supplied in adequate quantities from food or generated by degradation of body proteins (Table 9.1). Ten non-essential amino acids are synthesised in the liver, muscles, kidneys, and

intestine. Only the synthesis of arginine from ornithine and the hydroxylation of phenylalanine to tyrosine are liver-specific reactions. There are two semi-essential amino acids.

The amino acid pool (600–700 g) is distributed among the musculature (80%), the liver (15%), and the plasma (5%). Protein synthesis uses 300–500 g daily, and 2 g are used for the synthesis of other nitrogen-containing compounds (e.g. purines, porphyrins, and pyrimidines); a further 120–130 g are degraded daily. The amino acid pool is maintained at a constant level: 70–100 g comes from the diet, 300–500 g from protein degradation, and 30–40 g from biosynthesis of non-essential amino acids. The essential amino acids released by proteolysis are recycled in the neosynthesis of proteins.

The degradation of essential amino acids occurs primarily in the liver – only the three branched-chain amino acids (isoleucine, leucine, and valine) are broken down almost exclusively

Table 9.1 Essential and non-essential amino acids. Standard abbreviations are given in parentheses

Amino acid	Conditions in which essential
Essential	
Isoleucine (Ile)	
Leucine (Leu)	
Valine (Val)	
Methionine (Met)	
Threonine (Thr)	
Phenylalanine (Phe)	
Lysine (Lys)	
Tryptophan (Trp)	
Semi-essential	
Histidine (His)	Infants, patients with uraemia
Cysteine (Cys)	Neonates, liver disease
Non-essential	
Alanine (Ala)	
Aspartate (Asp)	
Asparagine (Asn)	
Arginine (Arg)	Critical illness
Glycine (Gly)	
Glutamic acid (Gln)	Acute illness
Glutamate (Glu)	
Proline (Pro)	
Serine (Ser)	
Tyrosine (Tyr)	

in the muscles. Non-essential amino acids are degraded in the liver and muscles (but also in other organs), mainly by transamination and oxidative deamination. The C skeleton, an intermediate product in amino acid degradation, is used for energy production in the citric acid cycle. Ketogenic and glucogenic amino acids are channelled into fat and carbohydrate metabolisms respectively. The amino group is excreted to a minor extent as ammonia.

The glucose–alanine cycle between the liver and the musculature is particularly significant. In muscle, ammonia is generated during the degradation of amino acids (particularly the branched-chain amino acids). The transfer of ammonia to pyruvate yields alanine, which is then transported to the liver (Figure 9.14). Here

the C skeleton of alanine is liberated for use in glucose synthesis via pyruvate, while the amino-N of alanine is incorporated as ammonia into the urea cycle. Up to 60–70% of the alanine released from the muscles is derived from glucose.

Amino acid metabolism is regulated by negative feedback, so that degradation and synthesis are kept constant. Only the branched-chain amino acids pass through the liver unmetabolised, irrespective of their concentration in the portal blood. Various hormones regulate the synthesis of amino acids and proteins: some inhibit protein synthesis, while insulin, somatotrophin, TSH, and glucocorticoids stimulate synthesis.

More than 100 plasma proteins are synthesised in the liver cell, the majority being glycoproteins. About 15 of the glycoproteins (including C-reactive protein, fibrinogen, haptoglobin, and ceruloplasmin) belong to the acute-phase reaction group. Numerous transport proteins, including albumin, haptoglobin, thyroxine-binding globulin, and transferrin, are also synthesised in the liver.

AMMONIA DETOXIFICATION AND ACID–BASE BALANCE

Ammonia (NH_3) is freely soluble in water, forming ammonium ions (NH_4^+). Ionised NH_4^+ is in a pH-dependent dissociation balance with NH_3. Alkalosis shifts the balance towards free ammonia. With a normal blood pH value of 7.4, more than 90% of the ammonia is available as NH_4^+. Most ammonia is formed in the colon; less is formed in the small intestine from glutamine. *Helicobacter pylori* also produces ammonium in the infected stomach. Twenty percent of the urea formed in the intestine is rehydrolysed to ammonium. The intestinal tract produces 300–500 mmol ammonia daily, and thus the concentration of NH_4^+ is 5–10 times higher in the portal vein than in the peripheral blood. The liver produces large amounts of NH_4^+ from the degradation of protein and amino acids, but this is directly detoxified in the urea cycle. Ammonium is also formed in muscle. In the kidney, 30–40 mmol/day of ammonia is produced

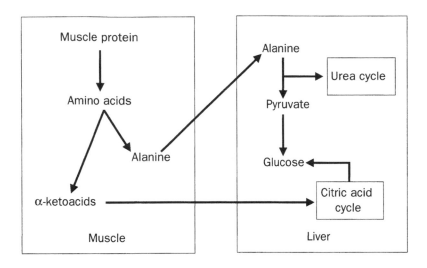

Figure 9.14 *The glucose–alanine cycle between liver and muscle.*

by tubular hydrolysis of glutamine and passed into the blood. The renal formation of ammonia is markedly increased by potassium deficiency and alkalosis. An increase in freely diffusible neurotoxic ammonia may result from a dissociation imbalance with ammonium and to inadequate detoxification of NH_3 and NH_4^+. The detoxification of ammonium takes place in the liver-specific urea cycle. Skeletal muscles and the brain detoxify ammonium via the glutamine cycle.

By far the greatest proportion of the nitrogen excreted by the body is as urea. In the urea cycle (ornithine cycle), ammonium and bicarbonate (CO_2) are converted in the mitochondria to carbamoyl phosphate (Figure 9.15). This enters the urea cycle, mainly in the periportal zone of the liver lobule. In the urea cycle alone, about two-thirds of the ammonia derived from amino nitrogen is irretrievably detoxified (definitive ammonia detoxification). One-third of the ammonia is trapped by the peripheral hepatocytes. By means of glutamine synthetase, glutamine is formed as a non-toxic transport form of ammonia. At the same time, glutamine activates the urea cycle (temporary ammonia detoxification). With increasing liver dysfunction, there is a marked loss of activity of the enzymes responsible for the urea cycle. Some of these enzymes are

zinc-dependent, and a decrease in enzyme activity occurs in zinc deficiency. Two moles of bicarbonate are required for the synthesis of one mole of urea. Approximately 500 mmol/day (~ 30 g) of urea is eliminated in the urine. Normally only about 25% of the capacity of the urea cycle is used. It is therefore virtually impossible for hyperammonaemia to result from isolated NH_4^+ hyperproduction alone. Alkalosis and hypokalaemia (caused for example by secondary hyperaldosteronism or the use of diuretics) shift the dissociation constant towards free, toxic NH_3. Thiazide diuretics in particular put an overload on the detoxification capacity of the scavenger cells, because a sufficient supply of bicarbonate for carbamoyl phosphate formation is unavailable due to the diuretic-induced inhibition of the mitochondrial carboanhydrase.

Glutamine constitutes the non-toxic transport form of NH_4^+ between the tissues. It is formed by the binding of NH_4^+ to α-ketoglutaric acid, which is converted to glutamine in hepatocytes, muscle, and brain cells. Glutamine synthesis and glutamate transport take place in the perivenous field, whereas the glutaminase reaction occurs in the periportal region.

The urea cycle localised in the periportal field requires a high concentration of NH_4^+. Through the glutaminase reaction, which is also localised

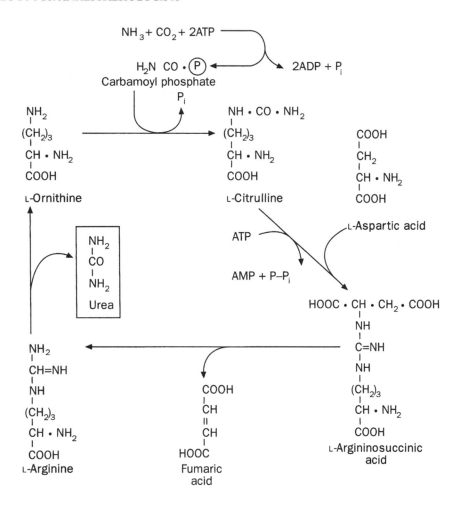

Figure 9.15 *The urea cycle.*

in the periportal field, an additional amount of NH_4^+ is released by glutamine splitting for the stimulation of urea synthesis. By contrast, glutamine synthetase has a high affinity for NH_4^+, so that even small amounts of ammonium that have escaped the urea cycle are 'temporarily' detoxified by glutamine synthesis in the perivenous blood. Only about 8% of the perivenous hepatocytes are needed for the fixation of residual ammonia.

In the kidney, glutamine is split by glutaminase into glutamate and ammonia; NH_3 is excreted in the urine. Glutamine is also released into the small intestine, where it is the main source of energy for mucosal cells. The liberated ammonia is transported as NH_4^+ through the portal vein to the liver for detoxification. NH_4^+ is rapidly converted into a non-toxic form: (1) by transfer to a ketonic acid with formation of a corresponding amino acid, (2) by formation of carbamoyl phosphate, and (3) by formation of the acid amide of glutaminic acid. The nitrogen from the acid amide group of glutamine remains in the metabolism for various syntheses. This group of acid amides is therefore called the ammonium storage group.

Large quantities of bicarbonate are constantly being produced in the body. The degradation of 100 g of protein yields approximately 1 mol (61 g) of bicarbonate. Bicarbonate neutralisation also takes place via the urea cycle, since the synthesis of 1 mol of urea requires 1 mol of bicarbonate. Besides the lungs and kidney, the liver thus plays an important role in acid–base metabolism and is partly responsible for pH homeostasis. The acid–base metabolism is influenced by the pH and HCO_3^- regulated switchover of ammonium detoxification from urea to glutamine formation: in acidosis, bicarbonate is conserved by curbing hepatic urea synthesis, whereas in alkalosis, bicarbonate is consumed by enhancing hepatic urea synthesis.

VITAMINS, TRACE ELEMENTS, AND METALS

Vitamins must be present in the diet. Only a few vitamins (e.g. vitamins A, K, B_1, B_5, B_{12}, folic acid and biotin) are formed in the intestine by bacteria. Plants constitute the main source of exogenous vitamins.

Water-soluble vitamins are readily absorbed under physiological conditions. They are transported to the intra- and extracellular fluid and act as coenzymes in a number of enzyme reactions in protein, nucleic acid, and energy metabolism. They are readily excreted via the kidney. Fat-soluble vitamins require the simultaneous presence of lipids and bile acids for their absorption. For transport to the liver, they are bound to lipoproteins in the chylomicrons. Fat-soluble vitamins are stored in the liver or fatty tissue. Vitamins A and D are secreted from the liver cells by means of carrier proteins. On undergoing biotransformation, fat-soluble vitamins become metabolically inactive as well as water-soluble and thus capable of being excreted. Vitamins participate in multiple ways in almost all processes of the intermediary metabolism taking place in the liver.

Trace elements are inorganic micronutritive bioelements and important components of enzymes, chromoproteins, and hormones. In humans, 15 trace elements are recognised as 'essential'. Deficiency or overdosage may have detrimental effects, since many trace elements are crucial to a variety of enzyme reactions. For instance, almost 200 enzyme reactions in the body are zinc-dependent. Fluctuations in zinc concentration are regulated by metallothionein. Other important trace elements are iron, copper (in blood 95% is bound to ceruloplasmin), selenium (in enzymes involved in free-radical scavenging and in the formation of triiodothyronine), manganese (manganese metalloenzymes), chromium (important for insulin action and involved in lipoprotein metabolism), cobalt (the central atom in vitamin B_{12} and its involvement in the release of renin and erythropoietin). Of the 4–5 g iron in the body, 65% is in haemoglobin, 10% in myoglobin, 5% in enzymes, and the remainder in storage compounds (47% in ferritin and 12% in haemosiderin) as depot iron in bone marrow, the liver, and spleen. The liver takes up iron predominantly from transferrin, formed mainly in hepatocytes (Figure 9.16). The liver plays a role in homeostasis of trace elements, and liver diseases may lead to persistent disturbances in their metabolism.

METABOLISM AND PRODUCTION OF HORMONES AND GROWTH FACTORS

Inactivation of hormones occurs mainly in the liver. Some are formed in or have their effect in the liver. Some hepatic effects of steroid hormones, in whose biogenesis cholesterol is involved, are shown in Table 9.2.

Conversion of 70% of the total T_4 (thyroxine) to T_3 (3,5,3-triiodothyronine) occurs in the liver. The metabolic effects of T_3 in the liver include an increase in protein synthesis, gluconeogenesis, ketogenesis, amino acid uptake, bile acid synthesis, biliary cholesterol excretion, and turnover of vitamin K-dependent clotting factors.

METABOLISM OF XENOBIOTICS AND ALCOHOL

Hydrophilic xenobiotics (foreign substances) enter the hepatocyte via transport systems using carrier proteins with no or only low substrate specificity. Lipophilic xenobiotics are much more common (about 70–80%) and rapidly reach the liver cells and organelles by non-ionic diffusion. As well as undergoing detoxification by the liver, metabolism of some non-toxic xenobiotics may result in the production of toxic

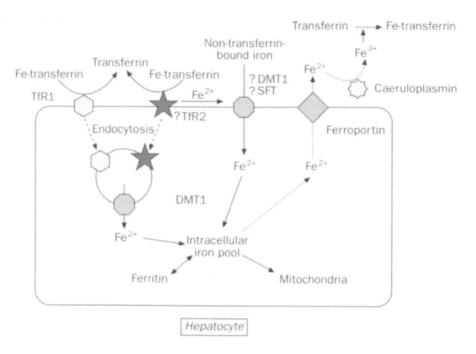

Figure 9.16 *Diagrammatic representation of the pathways of uptake of transferrin-bound iron and non-transferrin-bound iron by hepatocytes (see text for explanation). TfR1, transferrin receptor 1; TfR2, transferrin receptor 2; DMT1, divalent metal transporter 1; SFT, stimulator of iron transport. From Trinder D et al. Gut 2002; **51**: 290–5, with permission.*

metabolites (Figure 9.17). Furthermore therapeutically active substances can be converted in the liver into inactive metabolites ('inactivation') and inactive compounds (prodrugs) converted into active metabolites, for example, the inactive COX-2 inhibitor parecoxib is converted in the liver to the active compound valdecoxib.

In biotransformation, lipophilic substances can be converted into water-soluble metabolites that are more readily excreted. This process takes place mainly in the liver, in the smooth endoplasmic reticulum and partly also in the mitochondria of hepatocytes. Biotransformation is limited by the hepatic blood flow (flow-limited elimination) and by the capacity of microsomal enzyme systems (capacity-limited elimination).

Biotransformation of xenobiotics takes place in two phases. In phase 1, reactive (polar) groups such as –OH, –COOH, –SH, and –NH$_2$ are inserted by one of three chemical processes: oxidation, reduction, or hydrolysis. In phase 2,

hydrophilic residues are added to these groups by transferases that catalyse the conjugation with an endogenous substance. The hydrophilic conjugated product is readily excreted in the urine and/or bile. The most common conjugating ligands are glucuronic acid, sulphuric acid, acetic acid, and amino acids (glycine, glutamine, and taurine). Sometimes only phase 2, and occasionally neither phase 1 nor phase 2, is required for the elimination of a foreign substance.

Oxidative enzymes, in particular the microsomal mixed-function monooxygenases, are the ones most commonly responsible for the breakdown of xenobiotics. They contain the haemprotein cytochrome P450, consisting of a complex of at least 30 isoenzymes (see Volume 1, Chapter 2). The reductive enzymes are localised both in the microsomes and in the cytosol. They trigger the enzymatic transformation of ketones, aldehydes, sulphoxides, nitro and azo linkages, etc. The intestinal flora also contributes to the

Table 9.2 Steroid hormones and the liver

Glucocorticoids
1. Increase in gluconeogenesis
2. Increase in protein synthesis
3. Regulation of amino acid metabolism:
   - increase in amino acid degradation in muscle tissue
   - increase in amino acid uptake by the liver
4. Improved efficiency of urea synthesis
5. Inhibition of phagocytic activity of Kupffer cells

Androgens
1. Increase in haem synthesis
2. Stimulation of specific protein syntheses
3. Increased activity of cytochrome P450
4. Decrease in hepatic fatty acid-binding protein (hFABP)

Oestrogens
1. Increase in hFABP
2. Increase in δ-aminolaevulinic acid with decrease in porphyrin decarboxylase
3. Increase in protein synthesis
4. Stimulation of phagocytic activity of Kupffer cells
5. Inhibition of cytochrome P450 subtypes
6. Increase in lithogenicity of the bile:
   - increase in cholesterol excretion
   - decrease in bile acid excretion
   - decrease in secretion of bile

Progesterone
1. Induction of haem synthesis
2. Limited stimulation of protein synthesis
3. Substrate-dependent (inhibitory or stimulatory) regulation of the cytochrome P450 complex

reductive metabolism of foreign substances.

Changes in the activities of enzymes involved in biotransformation may be caused by various factors: (1) enzyme induction, (2) enzyme inhibition, (3) activation of an inactive enzyme, and (4) reduction in enzyme breakdown. Of these, enzyme induction is of the most important, resulting in increased drug metabolism and reduced pharmacological effect. The opposite occurs with enzyme inhibition. Many drugs and other substances (e.g. alcohol and smoking) cause changes in enzyme activity (see Volume 1, Chapter 18).

Alcohol uptake and degradation

Small amounts of alcohol may be formed in the body by intermediary metabolism, by some intestinal bacteria, and by endogenous intestinal fermentation when there is an excessive supply of carbohydrates in the food. About 20–30% of alcohol from oral consumption is absorbed in the stomach and 70–80% in the duodenum and upper small intestine. Five minutes after its uptake, alcohol is detectable in the blood, and maximum concentrations are reached after 30–60 minutes. Degradation is relatively slow, and accumulation, even at toxic levels, may therefore readily occur. When a diffusion balance has been achieved between the blood and the tissues (after 45–90 minutes), the alcohol concentration in the blood is 1.3 times that in tissues. The caloric value of alcohol is 7.1 cal/g (29.7 kJ/g). Approximately 75% (in alcohol intoxication, 85% and more) of the hepatocyte oxygen uptake is used for the oxidative metabolisation of alcohol, leading towards relative hypoxia of hepatocytes.

Three enzyme systems in liver cells metabolise 90% of ethanol to acetaldehyde; less than 10% is metabolised in the stomach by gastric alcohol dehydrogenase (ADH). About 5% is eliminated unchanged via the lungs and the skin, and 1% is excreted in the urine. The lethal alcohol concentration is 100–175 mmol/ml; the lethal dose is 2.5–3.5 g/kg (1 unit of alcohol is equivalent to 8 g ethanol).

Alcohol dehydrogenase

ADH is a zinc-dependent enzyme with five isoenzymes (ADH_{1-5}). Flushing syndrome in East Asians is based on an atypical $ADH_{2.2}$ and genetic reduction in the ADH_1 isoenzyme. Saturation of ADH occurs at a blood alcohol concentration of 10 mmol/ml (intoxication occurs at ~32 mmol/ml). ADH is not induced by chronic alcohol consumption. Higher alcohol concentrations, as well as protein deficiency, zinc deficiency, and sex and thyroid hormones, may decrease ADH activity. ADH catalyses the transfer of hydrogen from ethanol to NAD^+ with the formation of acetaldehyde. The toxic acetaldehyde is converted in the mitochondria

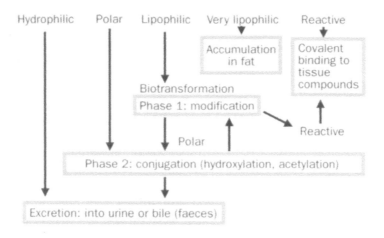

Figure 9.17 *Metabolism of xenobiotics.*

by aldehyde dehydrogenase (ALDH) to acetic acid, which is released into the blood and then converted in extrahepatic tissues to acetyl-CoA. This is utilised in the citric acid and fatty acid cycles as well as in cholesterol synthesis, or is oxidised to CO_2.

The microsomal ethanol-oxidising system (MEOS)

This is responsible for 10–20% of alcohol degradation. It is localised in the endoplasmic reticulum, predominantly in perivenous hepatocytes. MEOS is induced by chronic alcohol consumption, so that both the degradation of alcohol and the metabolism of foreign substances (and drugs) are accelerated with regular alcohol ingestion. Alcohol and drugs compete for the MEOS. Thus, alcohol consumers have an increased metabolising capacity for xenobiotics when sober (higher dose tolerance), whereas the breakdown of xenobiotics is slowed down under alcohol consumption (higher dose sensitivity). Enzyme induction occurs at the earliest after 2–3 days of alcohol intake, persisting for up to 3 weeks after discontinuation.

Catalase

In the peroxisomes, catalase causes splitting of

hydrogen peroxide into oxygen and water, and can also degrade alcohol to acetaldehyde at alcohol concentrations above 20 mmol/ml.

IMMUNOLOGICAL FUNCTIONS

The reticuloendothelial system (RES) is a widely distributed cellular functional system, composed of sessile and circulating macrophages of mesenchymal origin, with phagocytic capability for particulate material. In the liver, they are present as sinusendothelial, Kupffer, Ito, and PIT cells. About 90% of the total RES is localised in the liver, where they filter, phagocytose, and metabolise foreign substances, and aid in the elimination of endotoxins. Sinusendothelial cells have a clearance function with respect to connective tissue macromolecules, fibrinolysis activators, bacteria, and viruses, as well as macromolecules and immune complexes. Hepatocytes are also able to eliminate antigens and immune complexes by means of their IgG-Fc and C3 receptors. Although the phagocytosis capacity of Kupffer cells is 14 times higher than that of hepatocytes, the liver nevertheless contains twice as many hepatocytes as Kupffer cells. RES cells and hepatocytes jointly form a strong barrier against antigens and immune complexes. The liver indirectly participates in humoral and cellular immune reactions by means of this phagocytosis of antigenic substances, and also of apoptotic cells. Bacterial lipopolysaccharides from the intestine are detoxified in the RES, especially by Kupffer cells but also by hepatocytes. There is a complex interaction between Kupffer cells and bactericidal neutrophils that migrate rapidly to the liver in response to infection. There is also efficient trafficking of dendritic cells from sinusoidal blood to lymph to promote antigen trapping and T-cell priming. Local presentation of antigen can also cause T-cell inactivation, apoptosis, and tolerance. Production of signal substances such as cytokines (e.g. interferons), acute-phase proteins, and eicosanoids (e.g. leukotrienes) is important in the interplay between various liver cell types and for the self-control of biochemical and biomolecular reaction cascades. Regulation of the cytokine balance partially occurs in the liver. Radicals and reactive oxygen intermediates have important immunological functions within the liver. Their action can also be detrimental to the liver, which is partially protected by anti-oxidative compounds such as glutathione.

FURTHER READING

Arias IM, Jacoby WB, Popper H, Schachter D, Shafritz D. *The Liver: Biology and pathobiology*. 3rd edn. New York: Raven Press, 1994.

Bass N. Organization and zonation of hepatic lipid metabolism. *Cell Biol Rev* 1989; **19**: 61–86.

Baumann H, Gauldie J. The acute phase response. *Immunol Today* 1994; **15**: 74–80.

Bircher J, Benhamou J-P, McIntyre N, Rizzetto M, Rodés J, eds. *Oxford Textbook of Clinical Hepatology*. 2nd edn. Oxford: Oxford University Press, 1999: 3–447.

Bismuth H. Surgical anatomy and anatomical surgery of the liver. *World J Surg* 1982; **6**: 3–9.

Bloomer JR. Liver metabolism of porphyrins and haem. *J Gastroenterol Hepatol* 1998; **13**: 324–9.

Boden G. Interaction between free fatty acids and glucose metabolism. *Curr Opin Clin Nutr Metab Care* 2002; **5**(5): 545–9.

Bodo A, Bakos E, Szeri F, et al. The role of multidrug transporters in drug availability, metabolism and toxicity. *Toxicol Lett* 2003; **140/141**: 133–43.

Bourke E, Häussinger D. pH homeostasis: the conceptual change. *Contributions to Nephrology* 1992;

100: 58–88.

Brusilow SW, Horowich AL. Urea cycle enzymes. In: Scriver CR, Beaudet AL, Sly WS, Valle D, eds. *The Metabolic Basis of Inherited Disease*. 7th edn. New York: McGraw-Hill, 1995:1187–232.

Burton BK. Urea cycle disorders. *Clin Liver Dis* 2000; **4**: 815–30.

Correia MA. Drug biotransformation. In: Katzung BG, ed. *Basic and Clinical Pharmacology*. 4 edn. Norwalk, CT: Appleton & Lange, 1995: 48–59.

Cynober LA, ed. *Amino Acid Metabolism and Therapy in Health and Nutritional Disease*. London: CRC Press, 1995.

Fausto N, Laird AD, Webber EM. Role of growth factors and cytokines in hepatic regeneration. *FASEB Journal* 1995; **9**: 1527–36.

Hansen TW. Mechanisms of bilirubin toxicity: clinical implications. *Clin Perinatol* 2002; **29**: 765–78.

Häussinger D, Lamers WH, Moorman AFM. Metabolism of amino acids and ammonia. *Enzyme* 1993; **46**: 72–93.

Havel RJ, Kane JP. Introduction: structure and metabolism of plasma lipoproteins. In: Scriver CR, Beaudet AL, Sly WS, Valle D, eds. *The Metabolic Basis of Inherited Disease*. 7th edn. New York: McGraw-Hill, 1995: 1841–51.

Jungermann K. Metabolic zonation in liver parenchyma: significance for the regulation of glycogen metabolism, gluconeogenesis and glycolysis. *Diabetes Metab Rev* 1987; **3**: 269–93.

Kuntz E, Kuntz H-D. *Hepatology. Principles and practice*. Berlin and Heidelberg: Springer-Verlag, 2001.

Kwiterovich PO Jr. The metabolic pathways of high-density lipoprotein, low-density lipoprotein, and triglycerides: a current review. *Am J Cardiol* 2000; **86**(12A): 5L–10L.

Lautt WW. Hepatic vasculature: a conceptual review. *Gastroenterology* 1977; **73**: 1163–9.

McClain CJ, Marsano L, Burk RF, Bacon B. Trace metals in liver disease. *Semin Liver Dis* 1991; **11**: 321–39.

MacSween RNM, Scothorne RJ. Developmental anatomy and normal structure. In: MacSween RNM, Anthony PP, Scheuer PJ, Burt AD, Portmann BC, eds. *Pathology of the Liver*. Edinburgh: Churchill Livingstone, 1994: 1–49.

Meijer AJ, Lamers WH, Chamuleau RAFM. Nitrogen metabolism and ornithine cycle function. *Physiolog Rev* 1990; **70**: 701–48.

Olde Damink SW, Deutz NE, de Jong CH, Soeters PB, Jalan R. Interorgan ammonia metabolism in liver failure. *Neurochem Int* 2002; **41**: 177–88.

Oude Elferink RPJ. Understanding and controlling hepatobiliary function. *Best Pract Res Clin*

Gastroenterol 2002; **16**: 1025–34.

Rappaport A. The acinus-microvascular unit of the liver. In: Lautt WW, ed. *Hepatic Circulation in Health and Disease*. New York: Raven Press, 1981: 175–92.

Roach PJ. Glycogen and its metabolism. *Curr Mol Med* 2002; **2**: 101–20.

Schaffer EA. Cholestasis: the ABCs of cellular mechanisms for impaired bile secretion; transporters and genes. *Can J Gastroenterol* 2002; **16**(6): 380–9.

Sternlieb I. Copper and zinc. In: Arias IM, Jacoby WB, Popper H, Schachter D, Shafritz D. *The Liver: Biology and pathobiology*. 3rd edn. New York: Raven Press, 1994: 585–96.

Trauner M, Boyer JL. Bile salt transporters: molecular characterization, function and regulation. *Physiol Rev* 2003; **83**: 633–70.

Trinder D, Fox C, Vautier G, Olynyk JK. Molecular pathogenesis of iron overload. *Gut* 2002; **51**: 290–5.

Wick MJ, Leithauser F, Reimann J. The hepatic immune system. *Crit Rev Immunol* 2002; **22**: 47–103.

Young SP, Aisen P. The liver and iron. In: Arias IM, Jacoby WB, Popper H, Schachter D, Shafritz D. *The Liver: Biology and pathobiology*. 3rd edn. New York: Raven Press, 1994: 597–617.

10

Immunology

Ilias IN Doxiadis, James G Bovill

INTRODUCTION

The immune system is an integrated host defence system, involving numerous cells and molecules, that defends the body against invading organisms, foreign antigens, and abnormal host cells (e.g. tumour cells). It is also actively involved in the rejection of transplanted organs and tissues and in a variety of autoimmune diseases. Immunity towards pathogens is crucial for the survival of the species. Over the million of years of coexistence with external threats from pathogens, animals have developed sophisticated defence systems (immunity) against these pathogens. In this chapter, a short description of the action of the immune system in humans is presented.

Humans have three lines of defence against the damaging effects of pathogens such as bacteria, viruses, fungi, and parasites. The first defence is the physical barrier provided by the skin and the mucosal system. While the skin is often considered as the main natural barrier, its overall area is small ($2\,m^2$) compared with the area covered by the mucous membranes that line the digestive and respiratory tracts (about $400\,m^2$). When these barriers fail to stop intruders, two different mechanisms are involved in the protection of the individual: innate (or natural) immunity and adaptive immunity. Innate immunity comprises the complement system, macrophages, and natural killer (NK) cells. The reaction of the innate immune system towards pathogens is relatively unspecific. Adaptive immunity is only found in vertebrates. As the name implies, the adaptive immune system can change to protect against specific invaders, i.e. it is pathogen-specific. The specific immune system 'remembers' past encounters with each pathogen or foreign antigen, so that subsequent encounters stimulate increasingly effective defence mechanisms.

INNATE IMMUNITY

Innate immunity is the primary immune defence system in a 'naive' individual, such as the newborn. It is the first line of defence against an intruder after the skin/mucous membrane barrier has been broached. It acts non-specifically but with a good efficiency. At the beginning of the 20th century, Bordier recognised that a system of soluble proteins found in the serum of any individual of a higher species complemented the action of antibodies towards a specific pathogen. This system was therefore named 'complement', and is composed of at least 25 different proteins that cooperate both to destroy invaders and to signal other components of the immune system. Like most other components of the immune system, the complement proteins are present in the blood in an inactive form. In essence, activation of any complement component requires the cleavage of a short polypeptide from the native protein, resulting in a 'long' polypeptide, which usually binds to the intruder's cell surface, and a 'short' polypeptide, which can act as an immune activator (chemoattractant). The proteins involved in the complement system are in general proteolytic enzymes, which activate each other step by step. Activation thus occurs in a sequential manner, each activated protein activating the next one in the cascade chain, in a manner similar to the coagulation cascade. There are three different complement activation pathways: the classical, the alternative, and the mannose-binding lectin (MBL) pathways. The main difference between the pathways is the manner of recognition of pathogens. After the initial activation, all three pathways follow the same route.

The classical pathway

The classical pathway is activated by a specific antibody (immunoglobulin M (IgM) and, to a lesser extent, IgG, but not IgA, IgD, or IgE) binding on the surface of the pathogen or non-self cells, a prerequisite being previous exposure to the specific antigen. This pathway is involved in type II and III hypersensitivity reactions to drugs. The starting point of the classical pathway cascade is the C1 protein, a large complex of three complement proteins. C1 is normally bound to an inhibitor protein, but when two or more C1 complexes come close together, the inhibitor is inactivated and the cascade is initiated, resulting in the formation of C3 convertase (see below). From this point, the classical and alternative pathways share a common final pathway (Figure 10.1). When antibodies react with antigenic material, the reaction leads to the exposure on the Fc region of the antibody of a binding site for C1 complexes, bringing them into close contact with each other, allowing activation of the complement cascade. Because IgM has five Fc regions, it is highly effective in complement activation. IgG antibodies have only one Fc region and are thus less effective than IgM. C1 does not bind to the Fc regions of other antibodies.

The alternative pathway

Activation of the alternative pathway requires binding of a complement component on the cell wall of the pathogen or endotoxins released by them. This pathway, which can be activated without previous exposure to the antigen (e.g. a drug), is involved in type I hypersensitivity reactions and anaphylactic reactions. The main event in the alternative pathway is the cleavage of C3, the most abundant complement protein to C3a (anaphylatoxin) and C3b (an opsonin). C3a stimulates mast cells to secrete chemical mediators such as histamine and leucotrienes, and can also directly stimulate smooth muscles. C3b, which is very reactive, attaches to the surfaces of microorganisms to facilitate their ingestion by phagocytes (opsonisation). It binds to two chemical groups (amino or hydroxyl groups) that are found on the cell surfaces of microorganisms. If binding does not occur within about 60 ms of C3a formation, it is inactivated by binding to a water molecule. Once bound, it interacts with two other complement proteins, B and D, to form C3 convertase. This is highly efficient at converting C3 to C3b, setting up a chain reaction or positive-feedback loop. C3 convertase also interacts with C5 to form C5b, which then combines with complement proteins C6 to C9 to form a membrane attack complex (MAC). This can open up holes in the cell wall of bacteria or multicellular parasites, resulting in their lysis and destruction. C3 can also be cleaved directly by thrombin and plasmin, the principal enzymes of the coagulation and fibrinolytic cascades, and by enzymes released by leucocytes.

Why does MAC not form on human cells? Fortunately, we have several mechanisms to prevent this. Human cells have a protein on their surface, decay accelerating factor (DAF), which accelerates the breakdown of C3 convertase. Yet another cell surface protein (protectin) removes MAC before it can make holes in the cell membrane. The blood also contain proteins capable of cleaving C3b to an inactive form.

The MBL pathway

This pathway uses the binding of the mannose-binding lectin to carbohydrates on the cell wall of pathogens as the activation step. Lectins are proteins, produced mainly in the liver, that bind to a carbohydrate molecule. MBL, as the name

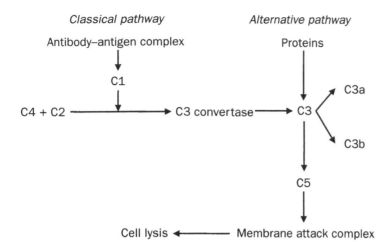

Figure 10.1 *The complement cascade of the innate immune system.*

suggests, binds mannose, a sugar found on the surfaces of many bacteria, viruses, yeast, and parasites. MBL, fortunately, does not bind to the carbohydrates found on healthy human cells and tissues. In the blood, MBL forms a complex with another protein, MASP. When MBL binds to the mannose on the surface of an invading organism, the MASP protein acts as a convertase, cleaving C3 to C3b.

Lysis of pathogens is only one role of the complement system. C3a and C5a, the short polypeptides cleaved from the native protein, act as chemoattractants that recruit immune cells such as T lymphocytes, macrophages, and other phagocytes to the site of infection. Components of the complement system also help to remove immune complexes from the periphery and transfer them to the spleen for elimination. The activity of the complement system is tightly controlled by an inhibitory system that prevents hyperreactivity, which might lead to lysis of the individual's own cells. The deletion or mutation leading to non-active inhibitor genes is one cause of some inherited diseases. Advances in the understanding of the complement system, and especially of its inhibitors, have made it possible to genetically modify animals, especially pigs (transgenic pigs), in which inhibitors of the human complement system have been introduced in order to reduce or abolish xenoantibody-mediated cell destruction after eventual transplantation.

The natural killer (NK) cell and its role in immunity

Until recently, only soluble components such as those of the complement system were attributed to innate immunity. Now, the bone marrow-derived NK cells are also thought to be involved in innate immunity. NK cells can be seen as the missing link between innate and adaptive immunity. They express a variety of receptors on their cell surface that can either increase the efficiency of killing (killer activating receptors, KAR) or inhibit killing (killer inhibiting receptors, KIR). NK cells are able to lyse cells not expressing self-proteins, mainly of the major histocompatibility complex (MHC), on their cell surface. They are the only cell type in the body able to recognise cells lacking the expression of self HLA class I molecules. These molecules, which are the main mode of transport of specific peptides to the cell surface, are the targets of viral infection. Many viruses encode proteins able to interfere with class I presentation of viral peptides to CD8+ effector cells, and this can reduce the immune response towards these viruses. Similar reduction or downregulation of class I antigen presentation also occurs in tumour cells. NK cells are the main defence mechanism that an organism has towards such attacks. In addition to killing virus-infected and tumour cells, NK cells also release a variety of cytokines that activate phagocytes and recruit T lymphocytes.

ADAPTIVE IMMUNITY

Innate immunity is primarily directed towards pathogens such as bacteria and fungi but is less efficient against another category of intruders, the viruses. Adaptive immunity plays the major role in protection against this type of pathogen, and also against other foreign invaders such as chemicals and drugs. The adaptive immune system, as the name implies, can change to protect against specific invaders, i.e. it is pathogen-specific. The specific immune system 'remembers' past encounters with each pathogen or foreign antigen, so that subsequent encounters stimulate increasingly effective defence mechanisms. This system also serves to amplify the protective responses of the non-specific, natural immunity. Specific immune responses take two forms: humoral and cellular immunity.

Humoral immunity

Humoral immunity is characterised by the appearance of immunoglobulins, or antibodies. These combine with the inducing substance (antigen) that stimulated their production. There are five classes of antibodies: IgM, IgG, IgA, IgE, and IgD. IgG and IgM are secreted into the blood and are known as soluble gamma-globulins. IgM is the first antibody detected after the prelimary exposure to an antigen, while IgG is the predominant one produced following secondary exposure, and is the immunoglobulin most abundant in normal serum. Other antibodiess, such as IgE, are cytotropic, i.e. they are carried to cells in the skin and other tissues, where they become fixed to the cell surface. They are normally present in the blood in only low concentrations. IgE binds almost exclusively to mast cells and basophils. Table 10.1 shows the functions of the various types of immunoglobulins. Protection mediated by antibodies can be transferred from one individual to another by serum or colostrum.

Antibodies have a Y-shaped structure, with four polypeptide chains (two light and two heavy) connected by disulphide bonds (Figure 10.2). The Fab fragments contain the antigen-binding sites while the Fc portion can bind to specific receptors (Fc receptors) on the surfaces of cells such as macrophages (Figure 10.3). The Fc region also binds components of the complement system.

Antibodies have two functions. One is to recognise and interact specifically with antigens that are foreign to the host. Most antigens are proteins, polysaccharides or lipid macromolecules with molecular weights over 5000 Da. Smaller molecules (e.g. drugs) are incapable of initiating an immune response unless they are attached to a protein. It is, however, the smaller molecule, called a hapten, that determines the antigenic specificity.

The second antibody function is activation of the host's defence systems. With the first exposure to an antigen (the primary response), antibodies can be detected after about 1 week, reaching a maximum at about 2 weeks. These

Table 10.1 Function of human immunoglobulin isotypes

Function	IgM	IgD	IgG1	IgG2	IgG3	IgG4	IgA	IgE
Neutralisation	Yes	No	Yes	Yes	Yes	Yes	Yes	No
Opsonisation	No	No	Yes	Variable	Yes	Yes	Yes	No
Mast cell sensitisation	No	No	No	No	No	No	No	Yes
Activation of complement	Yes	No	Yes	No	Yes	No	Yes	No
Transport across epithelium	Yes	No	Yes	Yes	No	No	Yes	No
Transport across placenta	No	No	Yes	Yes	Yes	No	No	No

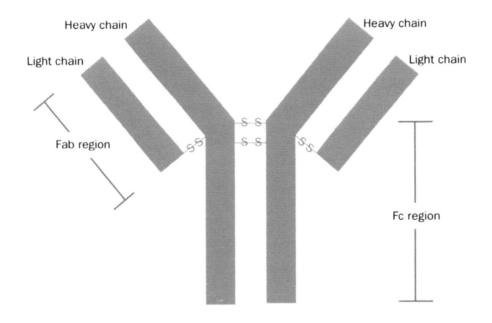

Figure 10.2 Structure of an antibody.

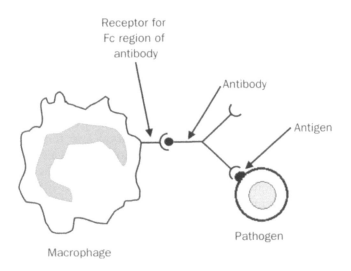

Figure 10.3 Antibodies form a bridge between an antigen on the surface of a pathogen (e.g. a bacterium) and a phagocyte (e.g. a macrophage), bringing the pathogen into close contact with the phagocyte and preparing the invader for phagocytosis.

antibodies are mainly of the IgM class. When a second exposure to the antigen occurs, a marked increase in the level of antibody can be detected after only 2 days, and the peak level, which is considerably higher than that associated with the primary response, is reached after about 1 week. A characteristic of secondary antibody responses is the production of IgG, IgA, or IgE class antibodies. Thus a primary response conveys both *specificity* and *memory* to the individual for that particular antigen.

Mast cells and basophils have receptors for

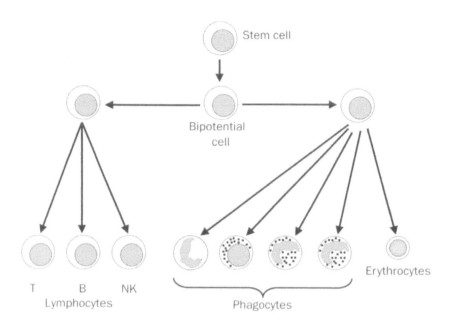

Figure 10.4 *Development of cells involved in the immune process from a haematopoietic stem cell in the bone marrow.*

IgE antibodies, which in certain circumstances attach to the membrane of these cells. Attachment of an antigen to the cell-fixed IgG antibody makes the cell secrete a range of active mediators such as histamine, leucotrienes, and kinins. This is the basis for some forms of allergic reactions, including anaphylactic reactions.

Cellular immunity

The key players in the cellular adaptive response are the lymphocytes, of which there are three main groups, B cells, T cells, and NK cells. Lymphocytes, and other cells involved in immune and inflammatory responses, such as monocytes and dendritic cells (specialised antigen-presenting cells), are derived from haematopoietic stem cells in the bone marrow (Figure 10.4). Unlike humoral immunity, cellular immunity cannot be transferred by serum but only by appropriately sensitised lymphocytes.

B lymphocytes and antibody production

B lymphocytes are responsible for the produc-

tion of antibodies. After maturation in the bone marrow, they migrate to lymph nodes and other lymphoid tissues. Within lymph nodes, antigenic stimulation causes follicles (local accumulations of lymphocytes) in the cortex to enlarge to form germinal centres. In the germinal centre, antibody-producing plasma cells are formed from B lymphocytes and migrate to the medulla. Lymphocytes within the lymph nodes migrate with the lymph to the blood and re-enter the lymph nodes via adhesion molecules on the postcapillary venules. There is thus a recirculation of small lymphocytes between blood and lymphoid tissues, and each lymphocyte may be exchanged between these compartments many times during its lifetime. In this way, sensitised lymphocytes originating from a local lymph node become widely distributed throughout the body.

Antibodies do not themselves destroy an invader, be it a pathogen or a foreign substance. Instead, they tag them for destruction by phagocytes, i.e. they opsonise (from the German 'to prepare to eat') the invader. When antibodies recognise their cognate antigen on the surface of a pathogen, their Fab region attaches to it, leaving the Fc region projecting. Phagocytes, such as neutrophils and macrophages, have surface receptors that attach to the projecting Fc region, so that the antibody forms a very specific link between phagocyte and pathogen (Figure 10.3).

Optimum antibody production requires cooperation between T and B lymphocytes. T cells responsible for cooperation with B cells are called helper T cells. They are involved in the switch in antibody production from the IgM class to the IgG and IgA classes. IgM antibody production is largely independent of T-helper cell activity. While still in the bone marrow B lymphocytes express a B-cell receptor (BCR) on the cell surface that recognises a specific region of an antigen, called the epitope. For a protein antigen this might be a region of several amino acids. Antibodies are very similar to the BCR, but are not anchored to the cell surface, and can thus be secreted into the blood. Each mature B lymphocyte produces only one kind of BCR and antibody, and is therefore specific for one antigen, called its cognate antigen. Fortunately, the cells are so diverse that collectively they can respond to millions of different antigens.

B cells must be activated before they can produce antibodies. Activation occurs in two ways, one involving helper T cells and the other independent of T cells. T-cell-independent activation involves the innate immune system. An important difference between the two methods of activation is the type of antibody produced; T-cell-dependent activation results in the production of IgG, IgA, or IgE antibodies, while T-cell-independent activation results in IgM antibodies. Once a naive or virgin B cell has been activated (initial activation occurs in the bone marrow), it 'remembers' its cognate antigen, and when it meets it again can rapidly proliferate (clonal selec-tion) and produce antigen-specific antibodies.

T lymphocytes

T cells, like B cells, are produced in the bone marrow and express receptors on their surfaces. Unlike B cells, which mature in the bone marrow, T cells mature in the thymus (T for thymus). Adaptive immunity is the result of teaching immune cells (T cells) to recognise and distinguish between self and non-self antigens. The role of the thymus is to select T cells whose receptors have specific properties: the T cell receptor (TCR) must be able to recognise the molecules of the self major histocompatibility complex (MHC) (positive selection) but not in such a way that they will be activated (negative selection). These two consecutive steps allow T cells that settle in the lymphoid system after maturation in the thymus to defend against intruders while avoiding autoimmunity.

Another major difference between B and T lymphocytes is that T cells only recognise their cognate antigens when these are presented to them by specialised antigen-presenting cells (APC). Three types of cells can act as APC: dendritic cells, macrophages, and activated B lymphocytes. T cells also only recognise protein antigens, whereas B cells can recognise any type of organic molecule. Helper T cells and suppressor T cells regulate the production and functioning of B cells, killer T cells (also called cytotoxic T lymphocytes, CTL) destroy cells that they recognise as foreign. These lymphocytes are also involved in a range of other immune responses, including delayed-type hypersensitivity and macrophage activation.

T lymphocytes express a variety of marker or 'co-receptor' molecules on their surface, which play important roles in recognising specific MHC molecules (Figure 10.5). Helper T cells, which express the CD4 surface marker, recognise antigens that are presented to them by APC in association with class II MHC molecules. They also secrete cytokines, low-molecular-weight proteins that activate macrophages, killer T lymphocytes, and B cells at sites of inflammation. Cytokines include various interleukins (IL-2α, IL-4, IL-6, and IL-10), tumour necrosis factor (TNF) and interferon-γ (IFN-γ). These are involved in the inflammatory process and also regulate the differentiation of leucocytes from haematopoietic stem cells. A summary of the different cytokines is shown in Table 10.2.

Cytotoxic, or killer, T cells express the CD8 surface marker and recognise antigens on the

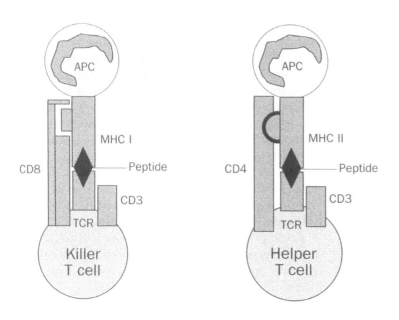

Figure 10.5 *Schematic representation of the presentation of a peptide antigen to two types of T lymphocyte. APC, antigen-presenting cell; MHC, major histocompatibility complex molecules; TCR, T-cell receptor; CD, cluster of differentiation marker molecules.*

Table 10.2 Effect of some cytokines on the immune response

Cytokine	Source	Effect		Haematopoetic stem cells
		B cells	T cells	
IL-2	Th0, Th1, some CTL	Growth, J-chain synthesis	Growth	NK-cell growth
IFN-γ		IgG2a synthesis	Inhibits Th2	Activates NK cells
IL-4	Th2	Growth	Growth	Growth of mast cells
IL-5	Th2	IgA synthesis	–	–
IL-10	Th2	MHC class II synthesis	Inhibits Th1	Growth of mast cells

IL, interleukin; Th, helper T cell; CTL, cytotoxic T lymphocyte (killer T cell); NK, natural killer; IFN, interferon; Ig, immunoglobulin; MHC, major histocompatibility complex.

surface of target cells in association with class I MHC molecules. They are especially effective at killing virus-infected cells. Cells that are infected by a virus signal this by expressing on their surface peptides derived from the virus together with class I MHC molecules. The peptide–MHC complex is recognised by the CD8 proteins of the cytotoxic T cell, which is enabled to kill the virus-infected cell, possibly with the cooperation of macrophages.

When the threat from a foreign invasion has been neutralised, most of the activated lympho-

cytes die. However, a subset of the antigen-stimulated B and T cells, called memory cells, remain. These do not differentiate into effector cells with the initial exposure to an antigen, but do express immunoglobulins on their surfaces. Memory cells survive for long periods (sometimes for more than 20 years) without further antigenic stimulation. They respond rapidly to a subsequent attack by their cognate antigen. Their development is crucial for the success of vaccination as a method of providing long-term immunity against infections.

MAJOR HISTOCOMPATIBILITY COMPLEX (MHC) AND ANTIGEN PROCESSING

The MHC, the most polymorphic system in higher vertebrates, is a region of genes encoded on the short arm of chromosome 6 that express glycoproteins, known as MHC molecules, on the surface of various cells. In humans, MHC molecules are referred to as human leucocyte antigens (HLA). They are expressed on the surface of most host cells, and are specific for that individual. Unless loaded with a foreign antigen, they enable immune cells to recognise their own host (self) cells. There are two types of MHC molecules: class I and class II. Both classes are very similar in structure, but they are differentially expressed on the surface of the different body cells. Class I molecules are expressed on almost all nucleated cells, class II molecules only on a few active immune cells, such as monocytes, dendritic cells, and activated B and T lymphocytes.

The principal function of MHC molecules is to bind fragments of foreign proteins, forming complexes that can be presented to T lymphocytes. Class I molecules (HLA-A, -B, and -C) present short peptides, and class II molecules (HLA-DR, -DQ, and -DP) longer peptides. The peptide-recognition region, capable of binding only peptide fragments of 10–20 amino acids, is a small cleft, like a basket, formed by two α helices and a floor. Between the α helices, and bound to the floor, peptides can be transferred from inside the cell to the surface for presentation. The small size of the 'basket' means that large protein antigens must be 'processed' to produce these smaller fragments that can bind to the MHC molecule.

Pathogens are pinocytosed in specific APC, the dendritic cells, and digested in specific protease-rich compartments. Immature dendritic cells express few MHC molecules on their surfaces. However, they become activated and mature after processing pathogenic proteins. Abundant expression of both class I and class II molecule–antigen complexes is the consequence. HLA class I molecules are loaded with peptides 9–11 amino acids in length and transferred to the cell surface. Class II molecules are loaded in other cell compartments than the class I molecules. The peptide length presented in these molecules is around 22 amino acids. After this processing, peptide-loaded class I and II molecules are transferred to the cell surface, where they can interact with T cells.

T cells are divided into CD4-positive (CD4⁺) (helper/regulatory/suppressor) and CD8⁺ (cytotoxic) lymphocytes, reflecting their effector capacity. The CD4 and CD8 molecules (CD: cluster of differentiation) are essential for binding of the antigen to the respective MHC molecules. The ligands of the CD4⁺ T-cell receptors (TCR) are class II molecules, while CD8⁺ TCR recognise class I molecules. CD4⁺ T cells are activated when they recognise the respective complex presented by the APC, together with additional co-stimulatory factors. This leads to the expression of the IL-2 receptor and production of IL-2, an autocrine (acts on same cell) cytokine that causes proliferation of the cells that produce it. These CD4⁺ cells in turn activate macrophages, B cells, and two subsets of helper cells (Th1 and Th2). Each subset of helper cells then produces its own profile of cytokines that control different immune responses. Naive CD8⁺ T cells can become cytotoxic effector cells via a strong co-stimulation activity provided by dendritic cells, or by additional help of CD4⁺ helper cells. Absence of co-stimulation leads to apoptosis (programmed cell death) of both T cell types.

Activated CD8⁺ killer T cells (cytotoxic) in the peripheral blood roll over the endothelium. When they find a class I molecule with a specific peptide matching their TCR on the cell surface, perforin and granzymes are secreted, leading to killing of the target cell. In addition, cytokines such as IFN-γ, TNF-α, and TNF-β are secreted. These are powerful activators of other players in the immune response. B cells are activated by Th2 helper cells that secrete IL-4 and IL-5 and express the CD40 ligand. Th1 cells activate macrophages via IFN-γ and other factors.

SELF-TOLERANCE AND AUTOIMMUNE DISEASES

Tolerance to self-antigens is a fundamental property of the immune system, which does not normally respond to the body's own tissues. Self-tolerance is induced and maintained by mechanisms that prevent the maturation or activation of lymphocytes, mainly helper and cytotoxic T lymphocytes that express receptors for self-antigens. This process of negative selection involves the specific recognition of these clones, which are deleted by apoptosis or inactivated during their maturation in the thymus. Tolerance to self antigens develops during fetal life by deletion of those T-cell clones that would have recognised self. Autoimmune disease results when there is a breakdown in the mechanisms that prevent the immune system acting against host cells. The patient with autoimmune disease must have HLA molecules that can present self antigens, and T lymphocytes with receptors that can recognise these presented antigens. Autoimmune diseases such as insulin-dependent diabetes mellitus, coeliac disease, multiple sclerosis, and lupus erythematosus are associated with specific HLA antigens, in particular HLA-DR3.

TRANSPLANTATION

Understanding immunity is important in treating autoimmune diseases and patients transplanted with an allograft, either a solid organ or haematopoietic stem cells. Specific transplantation immunology has been developed. Terms such as direct and indirect antigen presentation are only used in the context of transplantation. Since an allograft expresses class I and class II antigens, the immune system of the transplanted patient can recognise these molecules directly (direct presentation). The TCR of the patient's effector CD8+ cells recognise the donor HLA antigens. Indirect presentation occurs when the patient's dendritic cells enter the organ and can now present the donor HLA peptides via the patient's self molecules. Through processing, the peptides of the donor are presented indirectly (indirect presentation). Patients have about 100 times more directly acting CD8+ effector cells than indirect presentation cells. The immunosuppressive therapy that is used, however, is primarily directed towards the direct presentation pathway.

ALLERGIC OR HYPERSENSITIVITY REACTIONS

Hypersensitivity is a term used to describe exaggerated or inappropriate immune responses. In 1970, Gell and Coombs described four categories of hypersensitivity reactions, and although many reactions are more complex and do not easily fit into one of these classifications, they are still widely used as a simple guide to the basic mechanisms involved.

Type I hypersensitivity (immediate or anaphylactic reaction)

This occurs when endogenous substances that are not themselves damaging (e.g. pollen and certain foodstuffs or drugs) cause the production of IgE antibodies that fix to the surface of mast cells or basophils. On subsequent exposure, the antigen binds to the cell-fixed IgE, resulting in degranulation of the cell and liberation of vasoactive mediators, including histamine, serotonin, bradykinin, leukotrienes and prostaglandins. The effects may be localised to the bronchial tree, causing asthma or laryngeal oedema, or to the skin, causing urticaria. Anaphylactic reactions are more serious generalised reactions that can be fatal. The most common clinical features of anaphylaxis during anaesthesia are cardiovascular (74%), cutaneous manifestations (70%), and bronchospasm (44%). Anaphylactoid reactions are clinically indistinguishable from anaphylactic reactions, but involve non-IgE-mediated release of mediators from mast cells, or complement activation. It does not involve prior sensitisation, and can occur on the first exposure to the triggering agent. Type I hypersensitivity causes a local wheal and flare reaction with skin testing in sensitised individuals.

Type II hypersensitivity (antibody-dependent cytotoxicity)

This involves IgG or IgM antibodies that bind to cell surface antigens, resulting in either activation of the classical complement pathway or mobilisation of cytotoxic leucocytes. The clinical picture depends on the tissue involved. Type II reactions are responsible for a variety of diseases such as myasthenia gravis, glomerulonephritis, autoimmune haemolytic anaemia and thrombocytopenia, and acute allograft rejection.

Type III hypersensitivity

This occurs when a drug or other exogenous substance forms antigen–antibody complexes that are deposited on host tissue cells, with local inflammation or complement activation. Examples of drug-induced type III reactions are serum sickness, allergic arteritis, granulocytopenia, and some forms of allergic nephritis.

Type IV hypersensitivity

This is a delayed cell-mediated allergic reaction that occurs hours or days after exposure to the antigen. It involves sensitised T lymphocytes, which produce cytokines causing local oedema and inflammation. Type IV reactions typically involve the skin. The best known example is the reaction due to *Mycobacterium tuberculosis* (tuberculin reaction).

FURTHER READING

Sompayrac L. *How the Immune System Works*. Malden, MA: Blackwell Science, 1999.

11

Physiology of the nervous system

Martin Smith

NERVE CELLS

The neurone

Neurones are highly specialised cells that receive, assimilate, and transmit information. The neurone has a cell body that maintains its functional and structural integrity. Fine processes emanate from the cell body and divide further into finer processes. These structures are known as dendrites and their complex network is the dendritic tree. The effect of the dendritic tree is to greatly increase the surface area of the cell body that is available to make contact with other neurones at synapses. The size and extent of the dendritic tree varies enormously, but some large cells in the brain can have up to 10 000 synapses. The dendrites are the area of the neurone where electrical stimuli are received and integrated. The cell body, which contains the nucleus, is connected to an axon along which nerve impulses are propagated. Neurones can conveniently be divided functionally into four areas: (1) a receptor zone where synaptic connections are integrated, (2) an area where nerve impulses originate, (3) the axonal process that transmits the propagated impulse, and (4) the nerve ending where synaptic transmitters are released. Diagrammatic representations of motor and sensory neurones are shown in Figures 11.1 and 11.2.

The resting neuronal membrane is permeable to both sodium and potassium (Na^+ and K^+) ions, but Na^+ ions are actively extruded from the cell by Na^+/K^+-ATPase, whereas K^+ ions are retained intracellularly by negatively charged proteins. The resting membrane potential is determined by the Nernst equation and for a typical nerve cell lies around -70 mV. A specialised type of cell, known as the Schwann cell, surrounds the axons of many neurones. These cells wrap themselves around the axon to form up to 100 layers of membrane known as the myelin sheath. Myelin is a protein–lipid complex that electrically insulates the axon membrane. Gaps occur in the myelin sheath every 1–2 mm and are known as nodes of Ranvier. Nodes of Ranvier are 1 µm wide and are effectively spaces between adjacent Schwann cells where the axon membrane is exposed. There is a high density of Na^+ channels at the nodes, and this is where the action potentials form during nerve conduction. Myelin alters the electrical properties of the nerve fibre and results in increased conduction velocity because the impulse effectively jumps from one node to another (see below). A nerve impulse can be activated in the neurone by a variety of stimuli, including electrical, chemical, and mechanical.

Action potential

A nerve impulse is a physicochemical process accompanied by electrical changes in the cell membrane, termed the action potential (Figure 11.3). During the transmission of an impulse, the intra- and extracellular ratios of Na^+ and K^+ ions

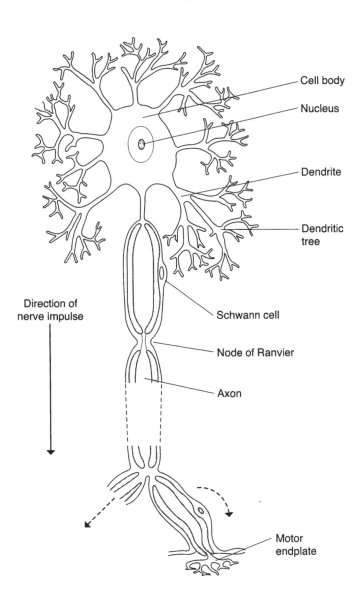

Figure 11.1 *Schematic representation of a typical myelinated motor neurone.*

Cell body

Nucleus

Dendrite

Dendritic tree

Direction of nerve impulse

Schwann cell

Node of Ranvier

Axon

Motor endplate

are reversed. Na^+/K^+-ATPase is inactivated during depolarisation and Na^+ ion permeability rises, allowing Na^+ ions to pass into the cell and the resting membrane potential to be changed. An action potential is triggered when depolarisation is sufficient for the membrane potential to reach a threshold value. Depolarisation of about $+15\,mV$ is usually sufficient to reach the threshold level and trigger an action potential. If the stimulus is of sufficient strength, an action potential of constant amplitude is generated irrespective of the strength of the stimulus. If the

stimulus has a subthreshold intensity, no action potential is generated. An action potential is therefore an all-or-none response. When the threshold potential is reached, a further rapid depolarisation to $+40\,mV$ occurs as Na^+ channels open. Na^+ ion permeability then begins to fall whilst K^+ ion permeability increases, causing a rapid and then slower repolarisation of the membrane. During repolarisation, the electrical status of the cell is restored by K^+ diffusing out of the cell. This allows repolarisation to occur more quickly than would be possible if it

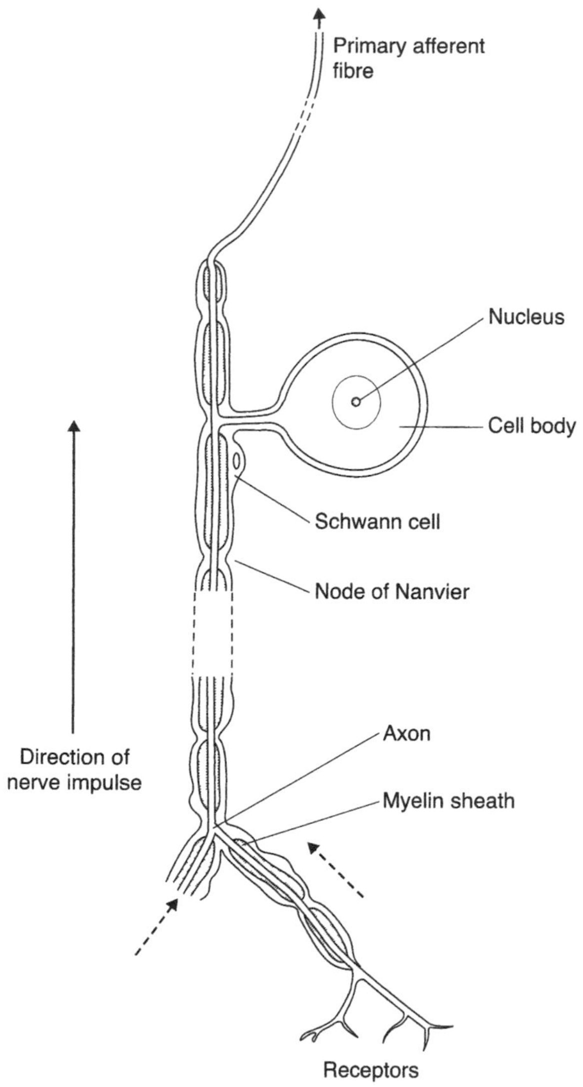

Primary afferent fibre

Nucleus

Cell body

Schwann cell

Node of Nanvier

Direction of nerve impulse

Axon

Myelin sheath

Receptors

Figure 11.2 *Schematic representation of a typical myelinated sensory neurone.*

depended only on Na$^+$ permeability changes. At the end of repolarisation, the resting membrane potential has been restored but the cell has effectively gained Na$^+$ and lost K$^+$. However, when Na$^+$/K$^+$-ATPase is reactivated, the normal intra- and extracellular ratios of Na$^+$ and K$^+$ ions are restored. Repolarisation is followed by a period of hyperpolarisation, after which there is a slow return to the resting membrane potential. The action potential persists for 2–4 ms, depending

upon the type of neurone. During much of the action potential, the membrane is unable to respond to further stimulation, and no matter how strong that stimulation the cell cannot generate a second action potential. This occurs because the majority of Na$^+$ channels are voltage-inactivated and cannot be reopened until the membrane is repolarised. This period is called the absolute refractory period. During the later part of the action potential, and for a brief

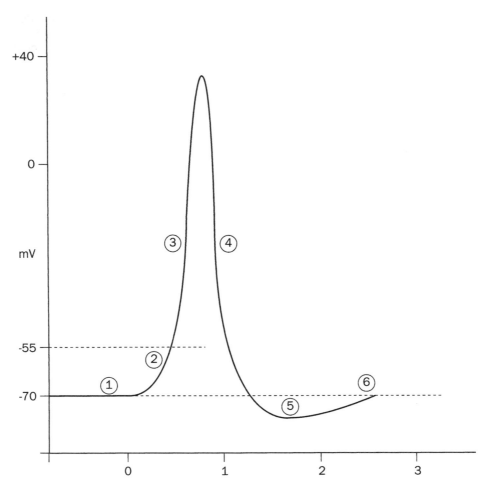

Figure 11.3 *Schematic representation of the motor action potential: 1, resting membrane potential; 2, depolarisation to threshold level; 3, rapid depolarisation; 4, repolarisation (rapid phase then slower phase); 5, hyperpolarisation; 6, return to resting membrane potential.*

period after its completion, the cell is able to fire a second action potential but a stronger than normal stimulus is required. This is the relative refractory period. It occurs because some Na^+ channels remain voltage-inactivated and a stronger than normal stimulus is required to open the critical number of Na^+ channels required to trigger the action potential. Permeability to K^+ remains elevated throughout the refractory period and contributes to its effects. The waves of depolarisation and repolarisation move longitudinally along the nerve membrane and result in conduction of the nerve impulse. Retrograde conduction of the impulse is effec-

tively prevented by the refractory period. In unmyelinated nerves, the impulses spread at speeds of about 2 m/s. Faster conduction occurs in myelinated nerves, where depolarisation can jump from one node of Ranvier to the next. Myelin is an effective electrical insulator and prevents flow of ions across the cell membrane. The breaks in the myelin at the nodes of Ranvier allow ions to move freely across the cell membrane at these points and allow the depolarisation to effectively 'jump' from node to node. This phenomenon, known as saltatory conduction, increases conduction velocity to around 120 m/s and is highly energy-efficient. Neurones can usefully be classified according to their diameter and speed of conduction (Table 11.1).

Action potentials in nerve cells are similar to those in other excitable tissues except for cardiac muscle, where a plateau follows depolarisation (Figure 11.4). This occurs because of entry of calcium into the cell, which has the effect of lengthening the refractory period.

Synapses

A synapse is a site where an impulse is transmitted from one neurone to another. There are two types: electrical and chemical. At an electrical synapse, two excitable cells transfer impulses by direct passage of electric current between them. This is enhanced by the presence of gap junctions that provide a low-resistance pathway for current flow between the cells. In chemical synapses, an action potential results in release of a transmitter substance from the presynaptic neurone into the synaptic cleft between the two cells. The transmitter diffuses across the synaptic cleft and binds to specific receptors on the postsynaptic cell, changing the potential of the postsynaptic membrane and initiating an action potential in the postsynaptic cell. Chemical synapses have a synaptic delay because of the finite amount of time required for passage of transmitter across the synaptic cleft.

Glial cells

Glial cells are non-excitable cells that are associated with neurones. In the central nervous system (CNS), there are three main types of glial cells. Oligodendrocytes are associated with myelinated axons and are involved in the production of the myelin sheath. They also form a structural framework to support the neurones and isolate them from each other. Oligodendrocytes store and transfer metabolites between small capillaries and neurones, and may be involved in the uptake and storage of transmitter substances. Microglia are small phagocytic cells that play a role in removing damaged cells. Astrocytes are larger star-shaped cells divided into two classes. Fibrous astrocytes are found extensively in the white matter of the CNS, whereas protoplasmic astrocytes are associated with cell bodies, dendrites, and synapses in the grey matter. Both appear to link nerve cells with blood vessels and are involved in the transport of nutrients.

Table 11.1 Classification of nerve fibres

Fibre type	Function	Myelinated	Diameter (mm)	Conduction velocity (m/s)	Spike duration (ms)
Aα	Proprioception, somatic motor	Yes	12–20	70–120	0.4–0.5
Aβ	Touch, pressure	Yes	5–12	30–70	0.4–0.5
Aγ	Motor to muscle spindle	Yes	3–6	15–30	0.4–0.5
Aδ	Pain, cold, touch	Yes	2–5	12–30	0.4–0.5
C – dorsal root	Pain, temperature, mechanoreception, reflex responses	No	0.4–1.2	0.5–2	2
B	Preganglionic autonomic	Yes	<3	3–15	1.2
C	Postganglionic sympathetic	No	0.3–1.3	0.7–2.3	2

BRAIN AND SPINAL CORD

The CNS comprises the brain and spinal cord.

The brain

The brain is composed of the brainstem, cerebellum, and cerebrum. The brainstem is the collective name for the medulla, pons, and midbrain. The medulla is continuous with the spinal cord and contains the lower cranial nerve nuclei, the gracile and cuneate nuclei of the sensory system, and vital centres for control of respiration, heart rate, and blood pressure. It is also the site of the decussation of the pyramidal tracts of the motor system. The pons connects the medulla to the midbrain and contains the nuclei of cranial nerves V, VI, VII, and VIII and the pontine nuclei. The brainstem is connected above to the deep structures of the cerebrum. The brainstem serves three main functions. It conducts motor and sensory signals between cerebral cortex/cerebellum and spinal cord via the reticular activating system, it is the location of the 12 cranial nerve nuclei (Table 11.2) and controls essential involuntary functions such as respiration, cardiovascular and gastrointestinal homeostasis. The reticular activating system projects widely to the cerebral cortex and limbic system and also has connections with many ascending and descending systems. It is responsible for generating the capacity for consciousness and the maintenance of circadian rhythms. The midbrain connects the pons and cerebellum to the hypothalamus, thalamus, and cerebral hemispheres. It contains the cerebral peduncles, whose ventral aspect becomes continuous with

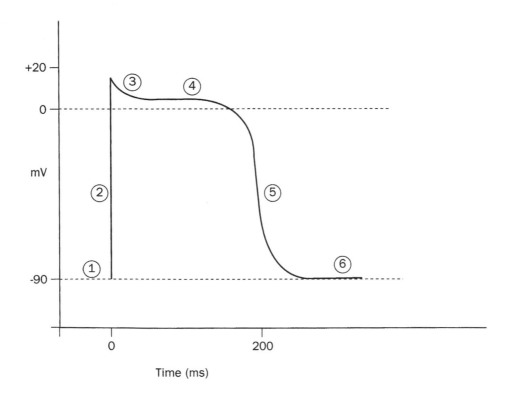

Figure 11.4 Schematic representation of the cardiac action potential: 1, resting membrane potential; 2, rapid depolarisation; 3, initial repolarisation; 4, plateau; 5, repolarisation; 6, return to resting membrane potential.

Table 11.2 Cranial nerves

Cranial Nerve	Function
I Olfactory	Sensory: smell
II Optic	Sensory: vision
III Oculomotor	Motor: extraocular muscles Parasympathetic: pupil
IV Trochlear	Motor: extraocular muscle
V Trigeminal	Sensory: face, cornea, scalp, dura Motor: muscles of mastication
VI Abducens	Motor: extraocular muscle
VII Facial	Sensory: anterior two-thirds of the tongue Motor: facial expression, periorbital muscles Parasympathetic: submandibular gland
VIII Vestibulocochlear	Sensory: hearing and balance
IX Glossopharyngeal	Sensory: posterior pharynx and tongue, taste Motor: swallowing Parasympathetic: parotid gland
X Vagus	Sensory: airway, ear, abdominal viscera Parasympathetic: heart, lungs, gastrointestinal tract
XI Accessory	Motor: sternomastoid and trapezius
XII Hypoglossal	Motor: tongue

the internal capsule. The dorsal aspect of the cerebral peduncles is the tegmentum, which contains the red nucleus, an important relay station in the complex pathways connecting cerebellum and spinal cord. The nuclei of cranial nerves II, III, and IV are located in the midbrain. The cerebral aqueduct runs through the midbrain and connects the third and fourth ventricles.

The cerebellum consists of two cerebellar hemispheres connected by the vermis, and communicates via the medulla, pons, and midbrain with the thalamus, cerebral cortex, and spinal cord. The cerebellum regulates fine motor control, posture, coordination, and muscle tone.

The cerebrum consists of the diencephalon and the two cerebral hemispheres. The diencephalon is the central part of the forebrain complex, comprising the hypothalamus and thalamus. The hypothalamus plays a vital role in control of the autonomic nervous system and endocrine systems and regulation of temperature, thirst, and hunger. The thalamus is a crucial area of the brain for integration of sensory pathways. The pituitary gland lies beneath the hypothalamus in the pituitary fossa and comprises anterior and posterior parts. It is connected to the hypothalamus by the infundibulum, which contains nerve fibres and the hypophyseal portal blood system that provides a direct communication between the pituitary gland and the hypothalamus. The two lobes of the pituitary gland have different functions. The anterior lobe contains cells that secrete growth hormone, prolactin, adrenocorticotrophic hormone (ACTH), thyrotrophin, luteinising hormone (LH), and follicle-stimulating hormone (FSH). Secretion of these hormones is controlled by the hypothalamus via releasing or inhibitory peptide hormones transported to the pituitary gland by the portal system. The posterior lobe of the pituitary gland secretes vasopressin and oxytocin.

The cerebral hemispheres comprise the cerebral cortex, the basal ganglia, and the lateral ventricles. The basal ganglia are discrete areas of grey matter within each cerebral hemisphere that play a role in controlling motor function. The major ascending and descending pathways to and from the cerebral cortex form the internal capsule that lies between the basal ganglia. The two cerebral hemispheres are separated by a deep midline cleft and are each divided into four lobes that are demarcated both anatomically and functionally. The frontal lobe is responsible for thinking, judgement, self-control, emotion, and other executive functions. The primary motor cortex, including areas for speech and eye movements, is situated at the posterior edge of the frontal lobe adjacent to the parietal lobe where the primary sensory cortex, responsible for sensory integration and association, is located. The central sulcus separates the main motor gyrus anteriorly from the main sensory gyrus posteriorly. The speech centre, known as Broca's area, occupies a small part of the frontotemporal region adjacent to Wernicke's area that is responsible for language interpretation. The temporal lobe contains the auditory cortex and areas for integration of auditory and other sensory input. The occipital lobe occupies the posterior tip of the cortex, and is responsible for processing of sight and control of complex occulomotor functions. Although the two cerebral hemispheres are of similar appearance and size, their function is not symmetrical. Almost all right-handed people have a dominance of the left cerebral hemisphere, but only 60–70% of left-handed people have right-hemisphere dominance.

The spinal cord

The spinal cord is continuous with the medulla and extends from the foramen magnum to the upper segment of the lumbar spine. Thirty-one pairs of spinal nerves are attached to the spinal cord by a dorsal sensory root and a ventral motor root. The cord is larger at the origin of the nerves to the limbs because of the high density of innervation to these areas. The cord has a central area of grey matter in the shape of the letter H that has 10 anatomically and physiologically distinct layers called the Rexed laminae (Figure 11.5). The dorsal horn is divided into six parallel laminae, with lamina I being the most dorsal. Laminae I–VI and lamina X are the sites where sensory afferent fibres synapse with dorsal horn cells and laminae II and III make up the substantia gelatinosa. Laminae XII–IX make up the anterior horns where α and γ motor neurones arise.

Reflexes

A reflex is an involuntary action elicited in a tissue or organ in response to a sensory stimulation. The reflex arc consists of a sensory organ and its receptors, the afferent neurone, one or more synapses in the CNS, the efferent neurone, and the effector organ or tissue. The afferent neurones enter the spinal cord via the dorsal roots or the brain via sensory cranial nerves. The efferent neurones exit the cord via the ventral root and the brain via the associated motor cranial nerves.

The simplest reflex arc is the phasic stretch reflex, of which the knee jerk is an example (Figure 11.6). Tapping the patella tendon stretches the quadriceps muscle, thereby stretching the muscle spindle and increasing the afferent discharge. In the spinal cord, the afferent fibre has a monosynaptic connection with the Aα motor neurone of the same muscle, resulting in rapid contraction of that muscle. No higher centres are involved. The sensory receptor involved in this reflex is the muscle spindle. This is an encapsulated structure present in, and parallel to, skeletal muscle. Muscle spindles contain several specialised muscle fibres called intrafusal fibres that

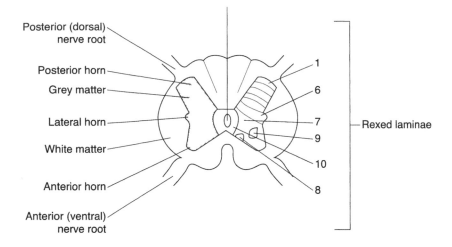

Figure 11.5 *Anatomy of the spinal cord. The H-shaped grey matter lies in the centre of the cord and is divided into anterior and posterior horns. The Rexed laminae are 10 anatomically and physiologically distinct areas within the grey matter.*

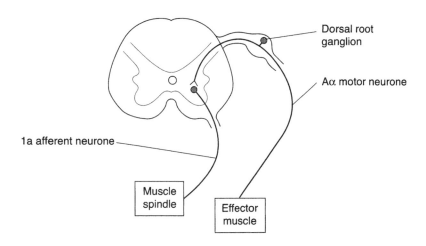

Figure 11.6 *Schematic representation of monosynaptic reflex. The knee jerk is an example of a monosynaptic reflex arc. Discharges in the 1a afferent neurone secondary to stimulation of the muscle spindle cause activation of the Aα motor neurone via a monosynaptic connection at the level of the spinal cord.*

are attached to the main muscle body (extrafusal fibres) or its tendon. Increasing the stretch of the muscle results in an increase in the rate of action potential discharge in the muscle spindle afferent fibre. Discharges in the afferent fibres can

also be activated by γ efferents when the muscle length is fixed.

The majority of reflexes are polysynaptic, allowing modulation of reflex actions via interneurones in the spinal cord. The synapse may allow forward conduction of the impulse, inhibition of the reflex, or modulation because of interaction with inhibitory and excitatory interneurones. The synapse allows convergence of these different effects onto a single motor pathway (the final common path). Widespread effects may therefore occur as a result of activation of a single reflex arc.

Muscle tone and posture

The tonic stretch reflex is a characteristic of antigravity extensor muscles whereby the muscle exhibits reflex tension when it is stretched. Stretch reflexes are responsible for muscle tone, which is the constant background muscle activity upon which body movements and posture depend. Maintenance of muscle tone and coordination of muscle movement requires simultaneous activation of α and γ motor neurones. A sensitive system transmits to the γ neurones information about the difference between the actual and desired length of a muscle to allow corrective action to be taken via a spinal reflex arc. Coordination of smooth and accurate movements depends upon a long reflex through the cerebral cortex, modulated by visual input, previous experience, and inputs from the cerebellum. Maintenance of posture also depends upon complex postural reflexes, including the supporting and righting reflexes. Supporting reflexes occur in response to changes in pressure distribution in various parts of the body and to contact with the ground. The reflex is initiated by stretching of interosseous muscles and results in increase in muscle tone around the vertebral column and in the limbs. Righting reflexes allow humans to stand the correct way up. They involve a complex collection of reflex arcs, including the labyrinthine-righting reflex, head and body righting reflexes, and other postural reflexes involving the cerebral cortex.

SPINAL CORD PATHWAYS

The locations of the major spinal cord pathways are shown in Figure 11.7.

Sensory pathways

Sensory impulses arise in the skin, muscles, tendons, and joints. The cell bodies of primary sensory neurones are situated in dorsal root and cranial nerve ganglia, and their central processes run with spinal nerves, through the dorsal root, into the spinal cord or with the appropriate sensory cranial nerve. Smaller fibres entering the cord terminate in laminae I or II and larger fibres in laminae III–V of the dorsal horn (Figure 11.5). Some fibres pass directly to motor neurones on entering the spinal cord and form a monosynaptic reflex arc, whereas others synapse in the dorsal horn of the spinal cord and influence the ventral horn via polysynaptic reflex arcs. However, the majority of sensory neurones join one of two major sensory pathways (Figure 11.8):

1. The posterior column–medial lemniscus system conducts proprioception, fine touch, vibration sense, and some autonomic fibres. The first-order neurones of this system turn medially after entering the spinal cord and ascend in the ipsilateral posterior column to the medulla, where they synapse in the gracilis or cuneate nuclei. Second-order neurones then pass to the contralateral side and ascend in the medial lemniscus to the ventral posterolateral nucleus of the thalamus. From here, third-order neurones project to the sensory cortex via the internal capsule.
2. The spinothalamic tract conducts crude touch and pressure (anterior spinothalamic tract) or pain and temperature (lateral spinothalamic tract). The first-order neurones synapse in the dorsal horn of the spinal cord (laminae VI and VII) with second-order neurones that cross contralaterally at the same level or at one or two segments higher. These then pass upwards in the spinothalamic tracts to the medulla, from where they continue as the spinal lemniscus to the thalamus. The spinal lemniscus also contains sensory fibres from the Vth cranial nerve. Third-order neurones again project to the sensory cortex.

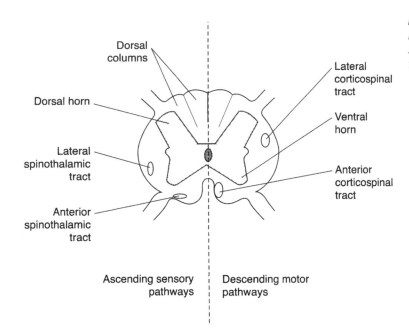

Dorsal columns

Dorsal horn

Lateral spinothalamic tract

Anterior spinothalamic tract

Lateral corticospinal tract

Ventral horn

Anterior corticospinal tract

Ascending sensory pathways | Descending motor pathways

Figure 11.7 *Diagrammatic representation of the principal sensory and motor spinal cord tracts.*

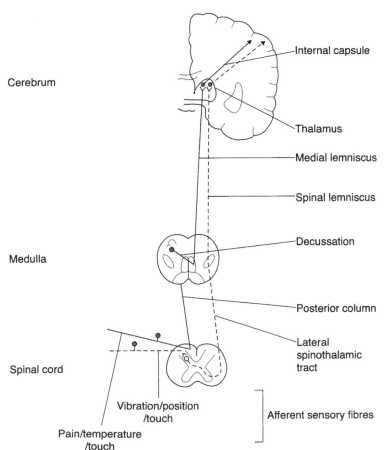

Figure 11.8 *Diagrammatic representation of the major sensory pathways.*

Internal capsule

Cerebrum

Thalamus

Medial lemniscus

Spinal lemniscus

Decussation

Medulla

Posterior column

Lateral spinothalamic tract

Spinal cord

Vibration/position /touch

Pain/temperature /touch

Afferent sensory fibres

Sensory pathways do not conduct impulses to the brain uninhibited, but are subject to intense descending control. At every synapse on the pathway, there is the opportunity for inhibitory or facilitatory modulation that results in reduction of irrelevant activity and improvement of discrimination. Some of the actions of the descending pathways may be related to the release of endogenous opioids. The thalamus acts as the major relay area for transmission of sensory inputs that ultimately become represented on the contralateral sensory cortex, which is the site of perception and appreciation of sensory stimuli, including pain. The major sensory area of the cortex lies within the postcentral gyrus, and areas of major importance, such as the hands and face, have a relatively greater representation.

Motor pathways

Upper motor neurones originate in the cerebral cortex and brainstem and run via the pyramidal or extrapyramidal tracts to lower motor neurones. Lower motor neurones, whose cell bodies are located in spinal cord grey matter and some cranial nerve nuclei, innervate voluntary muscle (Figure 11.9):

1. The pyramidal tract originates from the precentral gyrus and premotor area of the cerebral cortex and controls movement. Areas of greatest importance, such as the hands and face, have the largest area of cortical representation. The areas of the body are arranged in sequence over the motor cortex, with the legs being represented at the top of the gyrus and the head at the bottom. The pyramidal fibres run via the internal capsule and pons to the ventral aspect of the medulla, where they form the pyramid. Ninety percent cross to the contralateral side and descend in the posterior part of the lateral columns of the spinal cord (the lateral corticospinal tract). The uncrossed fibres pass down via the anterior corticospinal tract and decussate within the spinal cord at the appropriate spinal level. Some fibres (corticonuclear tract) also pass first to the motor nuclei of cranial nerves III–VII, IX, and X. Most fibres within the pyramidal tract synapse with intermediate neurones. The pyramidal tract is concerned with control of voluntary muscle, especially in relation to fine movements.

2. The extrapyramidal system is a less well-defined series of tracts connecting several areas of the premotor cerebral cortex with subcortical and brainstem nuclei. The extrapyramidal tracts descend from the lower brainstem as the rubroreticulospinal and vestibulospinal tracts, and pass with pyramidal fibres to interneurones in the spinal cord. Together with the pyramidal and sensory systems, they influence the lower motor neurones via reflex arcs. The extrapyramidal system is concerned with regulation of muscle tone and posture. It is mainly inhibitory, so that reductions in extrapyramidal activity result in increased muscle tone, spasticity, and uncontrolled tremor or movement.

Cerebellar pathways

Afferent pathways reach the cerebellum via the main ascending pathways in the spinal cord and transmit information from muscle spindles, Golgi tendon organs, and other proprioceptors. Efferent fibres originate in Purkinje cells in the cerebellum and cross to the opposite side in the lower half of the midbrain. From there, they project to the cerebral cortex and brainstem and to other nuclei such as the red nucleus.

SENSORY SYSTEM

Receptors

The sensory system includes the special senses, visceral sensation, and general somatic sensation. The latter includes exteroreceptive receptors in the skin that provide information about the external environment and proprioceptive receptors in muscles, tendons, and joints that provide information about muscle tone, body position, and movement. Receptors may be classified according to their function into mechanoreceptors, thermoreceptors, chemoreceptors, photoreceptors, and nocioceptors. Nocioception

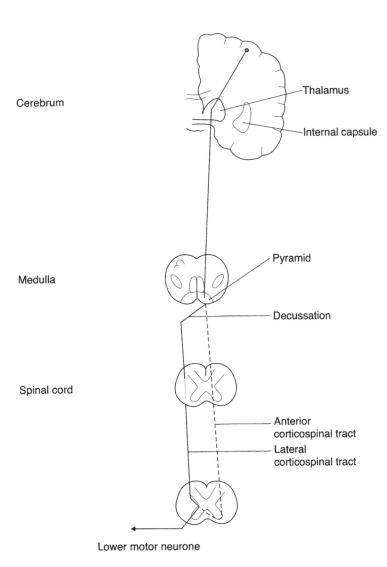

Figure 11.9 *Diagrammatic representation of the major motor pathways.*

Cerebrum

Thalamus

Internal capsule

Medulla

Pyramid

Decussation

Spinal cord

Anterior corticospinal tract

Lateral corticospinal tract

Lower motor neurone

is associated with free nerve endings, whereas other sensations are associated with encapsulated nerve endings specialised to one form of sensory recognition. Meissner's corpuscles sense touch, Ruffini's corpuscles joint position, and Pacinian corpuscles vibration and joint position. Receptors are sensitive to one type of stimulus or energy, and activation of the associated nerve results in awareness of that sensation in the brain. The nature of the sensation depends upon certain properties of the receptor, including its sensitivity, the intensity and nature of the stimulation, and receptor adaptation. The area of stimulation and number of receptors activated

also affect the perceived sensation. Sensory nerve fibres exhibit an all-or-none response, and therefore the number of neurones being activated and the frequency of the impulses are the only variables. Sustained receptor stimulation produces only a transient response because of processing at the level of the receptor. This ensures that the brain is not bombarded constantly by information when the stimulus is unchanging but is only informed of a change in stimulus intensity.

The modalities of cutaneous sensation are touch, temperature, and pain. Touch provides information on shape, texture, hardness, and wetness. Touch sensation is punctate in distribution, and deformation rather than pressure produces the stimulus. The smallest degree of deformation required to elicit a sensation varies from one part of the body surface to another. Sensory innervation is highest around hair follicles, where a complex nerve network is present around each hair root. Afferent fibres innervating touch receptors have a large receptive field. Touch sensation shows adaptation, exquisite localisation (dependent upon previous experience), and two-point discrimination. The skin is able to discriminate between warm and cold because of separate populations of receptors. Areas sensitive to cold are more numerous and the distribution may vary from day to day. The sensitivity of the skin to temperature varies from place to place, but the forearm is able to detect a temperature difference of as little as 0.2°C.

Nociception

Pain is an unpleasant sensation produced by stimulation of pain receptors (nociceptors) in free nerve endings. The initial stimulation is mechanical distortion of the nerve terminal, and this leads to an increase in the local concentration of K^+ and H^+ ions. Nociceptors have a high stimulation threshold for activation. They are distributed in a punctate fashion and are not related to receptors associated with touch and temperature. Pain is a perceptual experience that is affected by emotional considerations such as fear, anxiety, previous experience, and psychological attitudes. Pain evoked by a brief stimulus is perceived as coming in two waves. The first is distinct, sharp, and gradually reduces in intensity after a few seconds. It is replaced by a persistent, diffuse, and burning or aching sensation. This biphasic effect occurs because pain sensation is transmitted by two distinct groups of afferent nerve fibres: Aδ and C. Aδ fibres are stimulated by mechanical or thermal stimuli of high or low intensity and mediate the initial distinct, sharp pain sensation. C fibres, on the other hand, are stimulated by high-threshold chemical, mechanical, and ther-

mal stimuli, and mediate the burning and diffuse pain sensation. The first type of pain serves to remove the individual from the source of the pain by involving rapid reflex and behavioural mechanisms. The second phase of the pain sensation serves to prevent further injury and tissue damage.

Pain can be divided into superficial, deep somatic, and visceral. Superficial pain is well localised and has a sharp, pricking, or stabbing quality that may be short- or long-lived. Deep somatic pain is not well localised and is often referred to a place distant from its source. Most viscera are relatively insensitive to pain, but stimulation of tension receptors causes visceral pain because of stretching or inflammation. Visceral pain travels via autonomic nerves and may be severe in nature. It is diffuse and difficult to localise and may be projected to a position on the body surface.

Tissue damage of any sort initiates changes in the pain pathways that affect the pain experienced by the individual. These changes occur at the site of the tissue damage (peripheral sensitisation) or in the dorsal horn of the spinal cord (central sensitisation). Peripheral sensitisation lowers the threshold for the perception of superficial pain and occurs because of the release of inflammatory mediators, such as bradykinin, serotonin, prostaglandin, and leukotrienes, following minor injury. Histamine is also released locally and results in the familiar 'triple' response of redness, wheal, and flare. The collection of these inflammatory mediators (the inflammatory soup) results in sensitisation of afferent C fibres. This means that the stimulus required to generate an impulse is greatly reduced. Central sensitisation occurs at the site of the synapse between the C afferent neurone and the dorsal horn cell in the substantia gelatinosa of the spinal cord. The output from dorsal horn cells may be increased or decreased by the action of other systems acting on the synapse. Central sensitisation results in an exaggerated response in dorsal horn cells from Aβ and C fibre input.

Afferent nociceptive impulses pass via first-order neurones whose cell bodies lie in the dorsal root ganglia and that synapse with cells in the dorsal horn of the spinal cord. Aδ fibres synapse with cells in laminae I and V, while C fibres synapse with cells in laminae II and III (the substantia gelatinosa). Some afferent neurones divide before entering the cord and send branches up and down the cord in the tract of Lissauer before synapsing with a dorsal horn neurone. The cells in the substantia gelatinosa only respond to noxious stimuli. Most second-order (dorsal horn) neurones project to higher centres by ascending several segments in the cord before crossing contralaterally and joining one of three major spinal systems. The majority ascend within the anterolateral columns (the spinothalamic tracts) to the thalamus. Others travel via the spinoreticular tract and terminate in the brainstem reticular nuclei or via the spino-mesencephalic tract to the periaqueductal grey matter. The fibres connect from these areas to the somatosensory cortex.

There are powerful internal controls at all levels of this process and further modulation from descending systems at the substantia gelatinosa. The gate theory of pain was developed by Melzack and Wall in 1965 in an attempt to explain the modulation of pain transmission. The substantia gelatinosa contains many interneurones that are involved in the modulation of pain transmission. Melzack and Wall postulated that Aα, Aδ, and C fibres are all activated during painful stimulation and that these impulses flow from the periphery to the brain via a 'gate' located in the substantia gelatinosa. This is influenced by other neural pathways that act either to 'open the gate' and allow the impulse to pass centrally or 'close the gate' and prevent passage of the impulse. It is now apparent that the situation is far more complex than originally suggested. Stimulation of C fibres by deep receptors causes release of substance P at the synapse in the substantia gelatinosa and allows transmission of the pain impulse to higher centres. Aβ fibres inhibit the synapse presynaptically (via GABA effects) and prevent onward transmission. Small Aδ fibres, from superficial receptors, project cranially via the spinothalamic tracts and cause serotonin-mediated descending

pathways to inhibit transmission of pain impulses beyond the substantia gelatinosa via stimulation of enkephalin-secreting interneurones. The central descending system of pain modulation arises in the limbic system and periaqueductal grey matter, and the descending fibres lie in the dorsolateral funiculus of the spinal cord. It selectively has an effect on pain transmission. Some of the effects of the descending pathways that modulate pain transmission may also occur because of release of endogenous opioids.

Special senses

Vision

The eye is the organ responsible for perception and transmission of visual stimuli. The aqueous humour is the fluid within the eye and is produced by the epithelium of ciliary processes in the posterior chamber. Aqueous humour is formed by a process of active secretion at a rate of 1–2 μl/min. Compared with plasma, it is nearly protein-free and has a higher Na^+ and HCO_3^- ion concentration. It flows over the anterior surface of the lens, through the pupil, and into the anterior chamber. It is removed into venous sinuses of the sclera and thence into veins within the sclera. The small resistance to drainage of aqueous humour maintains an intraocular pressure of 10–20 mmHg. Aqueous humour has a mechanical and physiological function. It keeps the eyes rigid and maintains the refractory surfaces of the lens. It also provides nourishment to the avascular lens and cornea and acts as a buffer for the acid produced by anaerobic metabolism of the lens. The lens is the structure that allows an external image to be focused on the retina. The iris is the pigmented screen lying anterior to the lens, and its inner margin forms the pupil that controls the amount of light entering the eye. Minute sphincter muscles, innervated by parasympathetic nerves with an origin in the IIIrd cranial nerve nucleus, control pupillary diameter. The preganglionic fibres travel via the ciliary ganglion, and the postganglionic fibres via the short ciliary nerves to the eye.

The retina is the area of the eye where photoreceptors receive the visual stimulation. It is a highly complex structure that is densely innervated with specialised cells. Photoreceptors are of two types: (1) rods, which are peripherally distributed in the retina, mediate monochromic vision, and function in poor light conditions, and (2) cones which are responsible for colour and bright light vision and appreciation of fine detail. Cones have their greatest density in the fovae centralis of the retina. Light passes through several layers of neurones in the retina (ganglion cells, amacrine cells, bipolar cells, and horizontal cells) before reaching the photoreceptors. Each receptor consists of two parts. The outer segment consists of a set of folded invaginations of the membrane containing a high concentration of photopigment. The inner segment contains the mitochondria and cell nucleus and forms a synapse with other cells in the retina. When light reaches the photoreceptors, it bleaches the pigment, which is coupled to a G protein called transducin. Following a complex series of intermediary steps, ion channels are closed so that the effective permeability to Na^+ and Ca^{2+} ions is reduced. This causes hyperpolarisation of the cell membrane. Photoreceptor cells constantly release glutamate, and hyperpolarisation results in a reduction of glutamate release. The photoreceptor cells are connected to bipolar cells that become depolarised in response to light stimulus of the photoreceptor. Horizontal cells are responsible for inhibition of certain types of stimuli. Amacrine cells form a link between rod bipolars and ganglion cells but their exact function remains unclear. The ganglion cells are the output cells of the retina and respond to light stimuli with spike discharges. They project via the optic nerve to two subcortical visual centres. The superior colliculus is concerned with eye movements and orientation to visual stimuli, whilst the lateral geniculate nucleus is concerned with the sensation of vision and projects to the cerebral cortex. The visual cortex is situated in the occipital lobe, but other cortical areas also contribute to visual processing. The right cortex receives information from the left visual field of each eye and vice versa. The fovea has a greater representation than the peripheral part of the retina.

Hearing

The ear is responsible for hearing and balance. The ear can be divided into external ear, middle ear, and inner ear. The external ear consists of the pinna and external auditory meatus, which leads by way of the auditory canal to the outer surface of the tympanic membrane. The middle ear is the cavity that extends from the inner surface of the tympanic membrane to the oval window, an opening into the inner ear. The middle ear contains a chain of ossicles, comprising the malleus, incus, and stapes, that connects the tympanic membrane to a membrane covering the oval window. There is a second opening between the middle and inner ears, called the round window, that is also covered by a membrane. The middle ear is linked to the pharynx by the Eustachian tube, which is opened at the pharyngeal end during swallowing to allow equalisation of air pressure on each side of the tympanic membrane. The inner ear is a cavity within the temporal bone that contains the cochlea and vestibular apparatus. The cochlea is the organ of hearing and contains the bony and membranous labyrinth. It is a coiled structure formed by a division of the bony labyrinth into two compartments partitioned by a part of the membranous labyrinth. The cochlea duct is a tube formed from the membranous labyrinth and contains endolymph, which has a high concentration of K^+ ions and is similar to intracellular fluid. The bony labyrinth contains perilymph, which has a similar constitution to extracellular fluid. The organ of Corti is the sense organ for hearing and lies within the cochlea duct along the basilar membrane. The organ of Corti is made up of hair cells, the tectorial membrane, and a framework of several types of supportive cells. The hair cells are innervated by primary afferent fibres whose cell bodies lie in the spiral ganglion and by efferent fibres from the cochlea nerve.

The external ear acts as a filter that allows passage of frequencies between 800 and 6000 Hz. The external auditory meatus conducts variations in air pressure generated by sound stimuli to the tympanic membrane. Pressure waves cause the tympanic membrane and the ossicular chain to vibrate at the frequency of the sound. The ossicular chain effectively transfers sound energy from an area of low impedance (air) to one of high impedance (fluid) in an energy-efficient manner. The tympanic membrane has a larger surface area than the oval window and, coupled with the lever action of the ossicular chain, ensures that there is effective transmission of sound stimuli to the inner ear. Oscillation of the basilar membrane in the inner ear causes the hair cells of the organ of Corti to be subjected to shear forces at their junction with the tectorial membrane. Shearing forces on hair cells in one direction causes the cells to become depolarised because of an increased conductance to cations. This receptor potential results in release of glutamate and produces an action potential in the primary afferent nerve synapsing on the hair cell. The difference in potential between the endolymph and the intracellular fluid of the hair cells is an important factor in the sensitivity of the auditory system. Cochlear nerves that innervate hair cells at different points along the length of the organ of Corti are tuned to different frequencies of sound. Branches of individual primary afferents from the cochlear nerve synapse in the cochlea ganglion and project to several brainstem nuclei, including the superior olive and inferior colliculus. The majority of fibres from the cochlea nerve cross the midline in the brainstem, and central projections pass to the primary auditory cortex. As in the visual system, several additional cortical areas contribute to auditory processing.

Balance

The vestibular system detects head movements and the position of the head in space and, in association with the visual system, is responsible for balance. It has two sets of sensory apparatus to detect angular and linear movements of the head. The vestibular apparatus is contained within the bony labyrinth, but its function is dependent on the membranous labyrinth. It is connected to the cochlea duct, contains endolymph, and is surrounded by perilymph. The vestibular apparatus consists of three semicircular canals that lie perpendicular to each other and are aligned to detect events in three dimensions. Each canal has a small dilatation called the ampulla that contains sensory epithelium with hair cells. The hair cells are embedded into the cupula, a jelly-like flap that runs across the width of the ampulla. Currents created in the endolymph in response to movement of the head cause the cupula to swing backwards and forwards and result in bending of the cilia. The cupula has the same specific gravity as the endolymph and therefore does not respond to gravity but only to rotation of the head. The vestibular apparatus also contains the utricle and saccule, which contain two types of sensory cells responding to tilting of the head. Each sensory cell has several stereocilia and a single kinocilium that gives polarity to the cell. Bending of the hairs alters the ionic permeability of the cells and causes opening of ion channels and intracellular entry of Ca^{2+} ions. Glutamate is the putative transmitter at these cells. Receptors fire spontaneously, and bending of the kinocilium one way increase the firing rate whilst bending in the other direction decreases the rate of firing. The cell bodies of the primary afferent fibres lie in the vestibular ganglion, and the fibres project to the brainstem via the vestibular nerve. Most terminate in the vestibular nuclei, but some end in the cerebellum. There are interconnections with the reticular activating system, the motor nuclei supplying the external muscles of the eye, and with the spinal cord. This enables vestibular control of eye and head movements and autonomic adjustments in response to vestibular activity.

AUTONOMIC NERVOUS SYSTEM

The autonomic nervous system is involved in the regulation of non-voluntary bodily functions such as control of smooth muscle, cardiac muscle, and glandular secretion. It is the controlling mechanism of homeostasis and is regulated by autonomic reflex pathways and central modulating effects. The cell bodies of efferent (preganglionic) neurones arise from the brainstem and spinal cord and synapse with afferent (post-ganglionic) neurones whose cell bodies are situated in peripheral autonomic ganglia. The afferent limbs of these reflex pathways include visceral and somatic afferent fibres. The central control of the autonomic nervous system arises in the hypothalamus, limbic system, and brainstem reticular activating system. The close association between the autonomic and central nervous systems means that sensory inputs affect autonomic function as well as impacting on voluntary behaviour.

The autonomic nervous system is divided into the sympathetic and parasympathetic nervous systems on the basis of anatomical, pharmacological, and functional differences. The sympathetic and parasympathetic nervous systems act continuously to adjust activity in the cardiovascular and endocrine systems and in the gastrointestinal (GI) tract, often by exerting reciprocal control.

Sympathetic nervous system

The cell bodies of the preganglionic sympathetic neurones lie in the thoracic and lumbar areas of the spinal cord (T1–L2) and its ganglia form the paravertebral sympathetic chain. The motor axons of the sympathetic preganglionic neurones leave the spinal cord in the T1–L2 ventral roots and pass from the spinal nerves via the white rami communicans to the paravertebral ganglion at the same level. The preganglionic axons may then synapse in that ganglion, pass through the ganglion in a caudal or rostral direction, and synapse at another level, or pass through the ganglion and continue with a splanchnic nerve to synapse in a prevertebral ganglion. The effect of this complex arrangement is to allow fibres from any segment to synapse throughout the entire sympathetic chain, including at levels above T1 (the cervical sympathetic ganglia) and below L2, as well as in the prevertebral ganglia of the abdominal cavity. Some preganglionic fibres also directly innervate the adrenal medulla. The sympathetic nervous system therefore has a widespread distribution that is reflected in its functional effects.

Acetylcholine is the transmitter released at preganglionic nerve endings and noradrenaline at postganglionic endings. The activity of preganglionic neurones is modulated by several other neuropeptides, including substance P, enkephalin, somatostatin, nitric oxide, and serotonin. Activation of the adrenal medulla by preganglionic fibres causes the release of adrenaline. The general effect of the sympathetic nervous system is to cause a generalised arousal, the so-called 'fight or flight' response. Stimulation of the sympathetic nervous system causes an increase in heart rate and blood pressure, with redirection of blood flow from visceral organs to skeletal muscle. The pupils dilate, the skin blanches, and the piloerector muscles contract. The sympathetic nervous system also regulates visceral function.

Parasympathetic nervous system

The parasympathetic nervous system is less widely distributed than the sympathetic nervous system, and the cell bodies of the preganglionic neurones are located in the brainstem (cranial nerve nuclei III, VII, IX, and X) and sacral spinal cord (S2–S4). The cranial parasympathetic preganglionic axons leave the brainstem with the appropriate cranial nerves and synapse in the cranial parasympathetic ganglia (III, ciliary; VII, sphenopalatine and submaxilary; IX, otic) or on ganglia near the target viscera (X). In the GI tract, the vagal preganglionic axons synapse with neurones belonging to the enteric nervous system. The sacral parasympathetic preganglionic axons are distributed throughout the abdomen and pelvis on ganglia in the walls of viscera. Acetylcholine is the neurotramsitter at both pre- and postganglionic parasympathetic nerve endings. Stimulation of the parasympathetic nervous system increases activity in the gastrointestinal tract and reduces cardiovascular activity.

Enteric nervous system

The array of nerve fibres and ganglia in the wall of the GI tract is often called the enteric nervous system. This extensive autonomic reflex network receives inputs from the sympathetic and parasympathetic nervous systems and coordinates GI function. Afferent neurones, postganglionic motor neurones, and interneurones are present in the enteric ganglia of the Meissner's submucosal and Auerbach's myenteric plexuses. Meissner's plexus controls the muscularis mucosa and intestinal glands, whilst Auerbach's plexus is responsible for the activity in the muscle layers of the GI tract.

Limbic system

The limbic system is an important regulator of autonomic function. It consists of part of the frontal and temporal lobes and associated deeper structures, including the hippocampus, uncus, amygdala, cingulate gyrus, hypothalamus, and midbrain nuclei. The functions of the limbic system include regulation of motivational state, aggressive behaviour, sexual behaviour, feeding, olfaction, and generation of emotions. These are all functions that are essential for survival of the individual and the species. The hippocampus is responsible for memory function.

CEREBRAL BLOOD FLOW AND METABOLISM

The brain accounts for 20% of basal oxygen consumption and for 25% of basal glucose consumption, despite representing only 2% of body mass. Whole-brain oxygen consumption is 3.5 ml/100 g/min or about 50 ml/min. The brain is a very vascular organ and receives 15–20% of cardiac output at rest. This equates to a cerebral blood flow (CBF) of 50 ml/100 g/min. Preservation of the functional integrity of the brain involves maintenance of ionic gradients and the synthesis, transport, and reuptake of neurotransmitters. These are all highly energy-demanding processes. In general terms, about 60% of the brain's energy requirements are used to maintain electrophysiological function and 40% for cellular homeostasis. Ninety percent of cerebral energy requirements are met by glucose, but there are no significant stores within the brain. If cerebral blood flow is interrupted, glucose supplies become exhausted after about 3 minutes and cerebral oxygen delivery is

immediately compromised. Reduction in CBF below 20 ml/100 g/min results in disruption of the electrophysiological functions of the brain and loss of consciousness. When CBF falls to below 10 ml/100 g/min, cellular homeostasis cannot be maintained. The cell membrane pump fails, Na^+ and Ca^{2+} ions and water enter the cell, which swells and dies. Because of the unique sensitivity of the brain to ischaemia, it has a degree of luxury perfusion that allows a lower oxygen extraction ratio than other organs. This means that the venous blood returning from the brain is still 60–75% saturated with oxygen.

Control of cerebral blood flow

The substantial demands for a continued supply of glucose and oxygen to the brain are met by maintenance of CBF within strict limits. Three principal mechanisms are responsible for the control of CBF. These are myogenic, metabolic, and neurogenic.

Myogenic regulation – pressure autoregulation

Pressure autoregulation is the phenomenon that allows CBF to remain constant despite changes in cerebral perfusion pressure (CPP). CPP is related to mean arterial blood pressure (MAP) and intracranial pressure (ICP) in the following manner:

$$CPP = MAP - ICP$$

Under normal circumstances, ICP remains unchanged and therefore pressure autoregulation is often described in terms of changes in MAP. Pressure autoregulation occurs because of an intrinsic characteristic of cerebral arteriolar smooth muscle whereby myogenic reflexes alter cerebrovascular resistance secondary to changes in intraluminal pressure. Reflex contraction or relaxation of the vascular smooth muscle maintains a constant CBF in the presence of changing CPP. Myogenic reflexes are sensitive to changes in transmural pressure and not to changes in flow. As the CPP rises the arterioles constrict, and as the CPP falls the arterioles dilate. The response begins within seconds of a change in

CPP and is complete between 10 s and 2 minutes. The normal MAP limit for pressure autoregulation is between 50 and 150 mmHg (Figure 11.10). Autoregulation is affected by pathophysiological states and also by volatile anaesthetic agents (Table 11.3).

Table 11.3 Factors affecting cerebral autoregulation

- Arterial hypertension

- Hypoxaemia

- Changes in P_{aCO_2}

- Increases in intracranial pressure or cerebral venous pressure

- Intracranial pathology

- Volatile anaesthetic agents

Metabolic regulation

(a) Flow–metabolism coupling. It has been known for over 100 years that in the normal brain CBF is closely matched to the brain's local metabolic requirements for glucose and oxygen – a process termed flow–metabolism coupling. This occurs because of a vasomotor response to changes in cerebral metabolism whereby an increased neuronal activity causes an increase in cerebral metabolic rate (CMR) resulting in an exactly coupled increase in CBF to that area. Sensitivity of cerebral arterioles to certain metabolites such as K^+, H^+, and lactate has been implicated as a mechanism for this effect, but there is no time delay in adjusting flow allowing for accumulation of metabolites. The precise mechanism of flow–metabolism coupling remains unclear, but acetylcholine, serotonin, and nitric oxide have all been described as mediators. Flow–metabolism coupling is the most important factor in the local control of CBF.

(b) Arterial carbon dioxide tension. Carbon dioxide is a potent cerebral vasodilator, and CBF changes linearly by about 30% for each 1 kPa change in P_{aCO_2} between about 3.3 and 10.6 kPa. There is no further increase in CBF above 10.6 kPa due to maximal vasodilatation (Figure 11.11). These effects are caused by changes in extracellular H^+ ion concentration and cerebrospinal fluid (CSF) pH, and occur rapidly because carbon dioxide is readily diffusible. H^+ ions do not cross the blood–brain barrier, but CBF returns towards normal after about 6 hours because bicarbonate buffering gradually normalises CSF pH towards normal.

(c) Arterial oxygen tension. It has previously been accepted that CBF is unaffected by changes in P_{aO_2} between 7.5 and 40.0 kPa. CBF increases rapidly when P_{aO_2} falls below 7.5 kPa and almost doubles when $P_{aO_2} < 3.0$ kPa (Figure 11.11). However, there is some recent evidence that the threshold for hypoxic vasodilatation may be higher than previously imagined and may occur when S_{pO_2} falls below 90%. The mechanisms whereby changes in P_{aO_2} affect CBF remain unclear, but may include a neurogenic effect mediated via peripheral chemoreceptors or a direct vascular affect secondary to local accumulation of lactate. Potassium and adenosine are also potent vasodilators, and increased concentrations are found locally during cerebral hypoxia. Nitric oxide is a potent cerebral vasodilator and, as well as being a mediator for flow–metabolism coupling, may play a role in the changes occurring secondary to alterations in P_{aCO_2} and P_{aO_2}. Breathing 100% oxygen causes a small reduction in CBF of the order of 10%.

Neurogenic regulation

Traditional teaching suggests that neurogenic factors have little influence on control of CBF, but it has recently become clear that they have a major effect. The cerebral vasculature has extensive autonomic innervation, with the highest density being around the great vessels. Constriction of cerebral vessels occurs because of sympathetic stimulation via fibres arising in the superior cervical and stellate ganglia. The neurotransmitters mediating this effect include noradrenaline, serotonin, and neuropeptide Y.

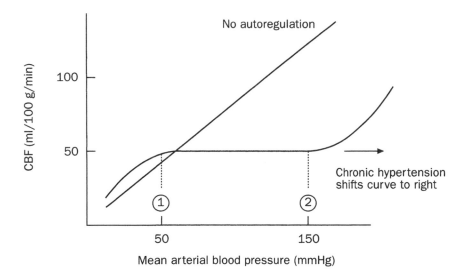

Figure 11.10 *Cerebral pressure autoregulation. Between points 1 and 2, cerebral blood flow (CBF) is kept constant because of changes in diameter of cerebral arterioles in response to changes in intraluminal pressure. At point 1, autoregulation fails because vessels are maximally dilated. At point 2, autoregulation fails because vessels are maximally constricted.*

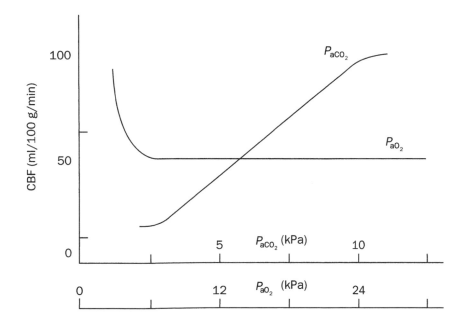

Figure 11.11 *Effects of P_{aCO_2} and P_{aO_2} on cerebral blood flow (CBF). CBF changes in a linear fashion with P_{aCO_2} between 3.3 and 10.0 kPa. CBF does not change until P_{aO_2} falls below 6.0 kPa.*

Parasympathetic stimulation causes cerebral vasodilatation via fibres originating in the sphenopalatine, otic ganglia, and internal carotid miniganglion. The neurotransmitters responsible for vasodilatation include acetylcholine, vasoactive intestinal peptide, and nitric oxide. There is also a sensory innervation arising from the first division of the trigeminal ganglion and from other somatosensory pathways originating in the thalamus. These pathways also cause vasodilatation mediated by substance P, calcitonin gene-related peptide, cholecystokinin, and neurokinin A. The cerebral vessels also contain opioid receptors that appear to modulate other vasoregulatory mechanisms, particularly under conditions of stress. It is likely that neurogenic factors produce rapid adjustment of CBF to metabolic demands and that chemical and metabolic intermediates are responsible for maintaining these changes. Sympathetic nerves have a role in the maintenance of CBF during hypoxaemia and hypertension, but the exact physiological role of parasympathetic nerves is less.

Blood viscosity

CBF is strongly influenced by blood viscosity, of which the haematocrit is the most important determinant. CBF does not change within the 35–45% haematocrit range, but increases when the haematocrit falls below 35%. The balance between oxygen-carrying capacity and CBF is optimal in terms of cerebral oxygen delivery with a haematocrit around 30%.

INTRACRANIAL PRESSURE

The intracranial pressure (ICP) is defined as the pressure exerted by the CSF in the lateral ventricles of the brain; in the normal adult, it is 10–15 mmHg. The ICP waveform is a modified arterial pressure trace with a superadded respiratory pulsation. Coughing and straining cause transient substantial rises in ICP even in normal subjects. The intracranial compartment consists of brain approximately 83%, CSF approximately 11%, and blood approximately 6%. Because the cranium is a rigid box, the volume of its contents

(i.e. brain, blood, and CSF) must remain constant if the ICP is to remain constant. This observation was first made by Alexander Monro in 1783 and has become known as the Monro–Kellie doctrine. The intracranial pressure–volume relationship is illustrated in Figure 11.12. If one of the components of the intracranial contents increases in volume, the other two can reduce to maintain a constant pressure (1 to 2 in Figure 11.12). At some point, this compensatory mechanism will fail as intracranial compliance becomes critically low, and then a small further rise in volume will cause a substantial rise in pressure (3 to 4 in Figure 11.12). Brain tissue is essentially incompressible, so any rise in ICP will cause CSF and blood to be expressed out of the cranium. The change in volume of one compartment to compensate for a change in another is known as spatial compensation. CSF plays the biggest role in spatial compensation because it can be expelled from the intracranial cavity into the 'reservoir' of the spinal theca. The majority of the intracranial blood volume is contained in the venous sinuses and pial veins. Reduction of cerebral venous blood volume is also able to play a role in spatial compensation and can be used therapeutically to reduce ICP in patients with head injuries.

CEREBROSPINAL FLUID

CSF surrounds the brain and spinal cord in the subarachnoid space. It acts as a supporting cushion and as a pathway for nutrients and chemical mediators. It is formed by active secretion, involving Na^+/K^+-ATPase and carbonic anhydrase, from blood in the choroid plexus of the lateral and third ventricles at a rate of 0.4 ml/min. CSF is a crystal-clear, colourless fluid that is essentially an ultrafiltrate of plasma composed of 99% water (Table 11.4). CSF circulates around the brain and spinal cord through the ventricular system and subarachnoid space. The lateral ventricles communicate with the third ventricle through the foramen of Monro, which joins to the fourth ventricle via the aqueduct of Sylvius. From the fourth ventricle, CSF circulates freely around the brainstem,

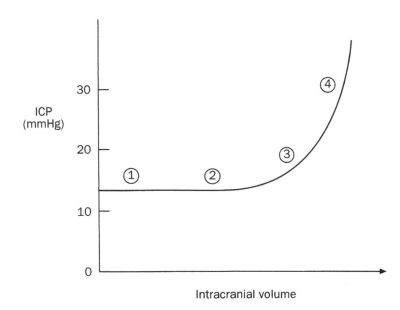

Figure 11.12 *Intracranial pressure–volume relationship. Between points 1 and 2, an increase in the volume of one component of the intracranial contents does not cause a rise in intracranial pressure (ICP), because of a compensatory reduction in volume of the other two. Between points 3 and 4, the intracranial compliance is critically low, and a small rise in volume causes a substantial rise in pressure.*

Table 11.4 Composition of cerebrospinal fluid (CSF) compared with plasma

	CSF	Plasma
Sodium (mmol/l)	144–152	136–148
Potassium (mmol/l)	2.0–3.0	3.8–5.0
Calcium (mmol/l)	1.1–1.3	2.2–2.6
Chloride (mmol/l)	123–128	95–105
Bicarbonate (mmol/l)	24–32	24–32
Glucose (mmol/l)	2.5–4.5	3.0–5.0
Protein (g/l)	0.2–0.3	60–80
pH	7.39	7.4

cerebellum, cerebral hemispheres, and spinal cord. The choroid plexus produces 450–500 ml of CSF each day, but most of this is reabsorbed through the arachnoid villi into dural venous sinuses to maintain a circulating volume of about 150 ml. The absorption of CSF is a passive process regulated by the pressure gradient between CSF and the venous sinuses. The production and absorption of CSF can be affected by many factors, including anaesthetic agents.

BLOOD–BRAIN BARRIER

It has become apparent that the blood–brain barrier (BBB) not only isolates the brain from the blood but also plays a pivotal role in maintaining the constancy of the internal milieu of the brain. Specialised tight junctional complexes between the endothelial cells of cerebral capillaries effectively eliminate gaps between cells and prevent free diffusion of bloodborne substances into the brain. A number of the proteins responsible for this barrier have been identified and the endothelium of the BBB is a complex and dynamic system rather than an inert barrier. The BBB plays a crucial role in transport of nutrients, neuromodulation, and osmoregulation. This is achieved by preventing entry into the brain of substances that could interfere with neurotransmission and also by regulating the transport of those compounds that are essential for the maintenance of normal brain function. Passage of substances across the BBB is predominantly a function of lipid solubility and the presence of active transport systems. The BBB acts as a semipermeable membrane that effectively maintains control of ionic distribution in the brain extracellular fluid. Sympathetic nerves protect BBB function, particularly during changes in arterial P_{aO_2} and systemic blood pressure. Four areas of the brain lie outside the BBB. These areas are collectively called the circumventricular organs and function as neurohumeral areas that allow substances secreted by neurones to enter the circulation directly, or as chemoreceptor zones where substances in the circulating blood can trigger changes in brain substance. The circumventricular organs are the posterior pituitary and adjacent median eminence, the area postrema, the supraoptic crest and the subfornical organ. The posterior pituitary gland releases oxytocin and vasopressin directly into the circulation and the area postrema acts as the chemoreceptor trigger zone that initiates vomiting in response to chemical changes in the plasma.

FURTHER READING

Fitch W. Physiology of the cerebral circulation. *Baillière's Clin Anaesthesiol* 1999; **13**: 487–98.

Iannotti F, Pringle A. Blood–brain barrier. In: *Neurosurgery – The Scientific Basis of Clinical Practice* (Crockard A, Hayward R, Hoff JT, eds). Oxford: Blackwell Science, 2000.

Inglis A, Fitch W. Physiology and metabolism of the central nervous system: anaesthetic implications. In: *Neuroanaesthetic Practice* (Van Aken H, ed). London: BMJ Publishing, 1995.

Menon DK. The cerebral circulation. In: *Textbook of Neuroanaesthesia and Critical Care* (Matta BF, Menon DK, Turner JM, eds). London: Greenwich Medical Media, 2000.

Moss E. The cerebral circulation. *BJA CEPD Rev* 2001; **1**: 67–71.

Roy CS, Sherrington CS. On the regulation of the blood supply of the brain. *J Physiol* 1890; **11**: 85–108.

Smith M, Crockard HA. The pathophysiology of the nervous system. In: *Essential Surgical Practice* (Cuschieri A, Giles GR, Moossa AR, eds). Oxford: Butterworth Heinemann, 1995.

12

Cell structure, function, and regulation

Yogen Amin

INTRODUCTION

All living creatures are made of cells. Cells are small membrane-bounded compartments filled with a concentrated aqueous solution of chemicals. Functionally, cells can be defined as objects that possess at least two major components of machinery for life: information transfer, which stores, distributes, reads out, and reproduces the information that controls the processes of life, and energy transduction, which changes energy from one form to another, stores it, and distributes it to execute the processes of life. All cells can be classified as belonging to one of two classes. Prokaryotic cells are cells that lack a well-defined, membrane-enclosed nucleus (prokaryote, from the Greek for 'before nucleus'); thus, the DNA material is not enclosed within a nucleus. Examples of prokaryotic cells include bacteria and blue-green algae (cyanobacteria). Today prokaryotic cells probably resemble the primordial cells from which all life on Earth was derived some 3 billion years ago. About 1.5 billion years ago, a second class of cells known as eukaryotic cells emerged that had a more complex internal structure than prokaryotes. Eukaryotic cells contain a nucleus (eu-karyote, from the Greek 'good or true nucleus') and cell organelles, which are semi-autonomous structures of defined function within the cell. Eukaryotic cells are as much as 10–20 times larger in diameter and thousands of times greater in mass than most prokaryotic cells. Organisms, which are made out of eukaryotic cells, are members of the kingdoms Protoctista, Animala, Plantae, and Fungi. To begin to understand the structure and function of cells as a whole, we now describe the various internal structures, that make up cells (Figure 12.1).

PLASMA MEMBRANE

All cells are enveloped by a cell membrane composed of lipids and proteins. This plasma membrane surrounds the entire cell and functions to regulate transport of materials into and out of the cell, coordinate the synthesis and assembly of cell wall, and receive hormonal and environmental signals that control growth and differentiation, amongst other functions. A lipid bilayer (Figure 12.2) forms the basic structure of the plasma membrane. The lipid molecules (primarily phospholipids, cholesterol, and glycolipids) are amphipathic, with a hydrophilic polar head group and a hydrophobic tail. The lipid molecules arrange themselves into bilayers with the hydrophilic head groups facing out, and the hydrophobic tails of the molecules facing each other within the interior of the bilayer. Proteins are embedded within the lipid bilayer, providing both structural integrity (by contributing to the cell's cytoskeleton) as well as cell function (Figure 12.3). Proteins that are present only on one or other side of the membrane serve primarily as enzymes, which activate or inactivate various metabolic processes. Glycoproteins found on the extracellular surface, together with

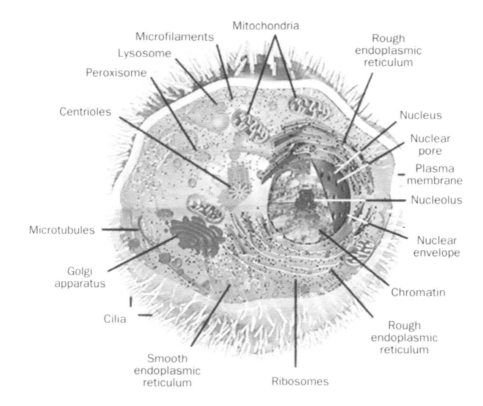

Figure 12.1 *Anatomy of the animal cell.*

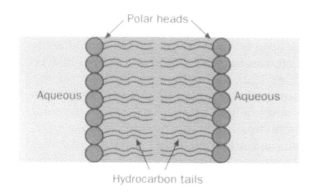

Figure 12.2 *A lipid bilayer.*

glycolipids, contribute to the glycocalyx (cell coat), a carbohydrate-rich layer that forms the outer coat of eukaryotic cells.

Some proteins span the entire membrane bilayer and are referred to as transmembrane proteins and include channels, carriers, pumps, and receptors. The channels allow small, water-soluble ions to diffuse across the membrane. Carriers actively transport materials across the bilayer, pumps actively transport ions across the bilayer, and the receptors, when activated, initiate intracellular reactions. Transport across the cell membrane occurs by diffusion, osmosis, active transport, and vesicular transport. Each of these will now be considered separately.

Diffusion

Diffusion can be simple or facilitated. Simple diffusion is a passive process by which uncharged particles in solution flow along a concentration gradient, from higher to lower, requiring no external source of energy. The rate at which material diffuses through a membrane is a function of its concentration gradient. The flux (i.e. the flow of a substance as measured by the number of moles of the substance that enters

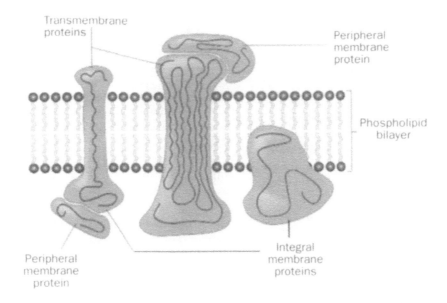

Figure 12.3 *Membrane proteins.*

a region in a unit time, e.g. a second) is proportional to the diffusion coefficient, the area of the membrane, and the concentration gradient, and is inversely proportional to the diffusion distance, i.e. the width of the membrane. The diffusion coefficient depends on the solute and the membrane through which diffusion is taking place. Lipid-soluble particles diffuse through the lipid bilayer of the cell membrane, and hence their permeability is proportional to their lipid solubility. Water-soluble particles diffuse through the aqueous channels formed by transmembrane proteins, and their permeability is proportional to their molecular size, shape, and charge.

Facilitated diffusion is a process that enables particles that are too large to flow through the membrane channels by simple diffusion to pass through bound to carrier molecules instead. This type of diffusion is responsible for the transport of glucose into red blood cells, muscle cells, and adipose tissue (in the presence of insulin). Again no external source of energy (or driving force) is required. The carrier protein undergoes repetitive spontaneous conformational changes during which the binding site for the substance is alternately exposed to the intracellular fluid and the extracellular fluid. The rate increases as the concentration gradient increases, until all of the binding sites are filled. At this point, the rate of diffusion can no longer increase with increasing particle concentration. This saturable process is governed by Michaelis–Menten kinetics.

Osmosis

Osmosis is the passive flow of water across a selectively permeable membrane down an osmotic pressure gradient. This gradient is created by the presence of different concentrations of solutes in the solution on either side of the membrane. It is related to the number of particles dissolved in solution, not their size, molecular weight, or chemical constitution. Hence, 1 mmol/l of glucose has the same osmotic concentration as 0.5 mmol/l of sodium chloride, as in solution the latter forms two particles. Changes in the plasma osmolarity cause cells to shrink or swell, as the osmotic pressure difference between the inside and outside of the cell causes water to flow out of, or into, the cell.

Active transport processes

There are two active transport processes – primary and secondary – and three carrier types – uniporters, symporters, and antiporters.

Primary active transport processes use the energy obtained from the hydrolysis of adenosine triphosphate (ATP, see later for further explanation of this important molecule) directly to transport material against an energy (concentration or electrical) gradient. The most common example of this active transport system is that of the sodium/potassium pump, which uses the membrane-bound ATPase as a carrier molecule. These pumps can be inhibited by drugs (e.g. digitalis) or if the concentration of the substrates that are required for its operation are too low (i.e. sodium, potassium, or ATP). Other primary active transport systems that rely directly on the hydrolysis of ATP to transport ions include the calcium pump on the sarcoplasmic reticulum of muscle cells, which maintains the intracellular ionic concentration below 100 nmol/l, and the potassium/hydrogen pump of the gastric mucosa cells.

Secondary active transport processes use the energy stored in the sodium concentration gradient to transport material against an energy gradient. Examples of this include the way in which glucose and amino acids are reabsorbed from the proximal tubules in the kidney and absorbed from the intestinal lumen by a sodium-dependent secondary active transport mechanism. Calcium is removed from the cytoplasm of cardiac ventricular (and other muscle) cells by a sodium-dependent secondary active transporter called the sodium/calcium exchanger; this mechanism causes muscle relaxation. The hydrogen produced by cellular metabolism is pumped out of the cells by secondary active transport, which is important for the maintenance of normal intracellular pH in all cells.

There are three types of carrier.

- uniporters, which are transporters of single particles in one direction, such as the facilitated diffusion of glucose;
- symporters, which transport two different particles in the same direction, such as the secondary active transport of glucose;
- antiporters, which transport molecules in opposite directions, such as the sodium/calcium and sodium/hydrogen exchanges.

Vesicular transport

Vesicular mechanisms transport many substances across the cell membrane by endocytosis and exocytosis.

In endocytosis, extracellular material is trapped within vesicles that are formed by invaginations of the cell membrane. The endocytotic vesicle pinches off from the cell membrane and then fuses with another intracellular vesicle (i.e. an endosome or lysosome), from which the ingested material is released into the cell.

In exocytosis, intracellular material is trapped within vesicles, which fuse with the cell membrane and are released into the extracellular fluid. Hormones, digestive enzymes, and synaptic transmitters are examples of this type of transportation across the cell membrane.

NUCLEUS

The nucleus is a 3–10 μm diameter structure, which directs all cellular activity by protein synthesis according to its DNA content. The nucleus is also responsible for transmission of genetic information to subsequent generation of cells. It is isolated from the cytoplasm by an envelope composed of two membranes. DNA is contained in the nucleus, packed into chromatin fibres by its association with histone proteins. When the cell divides, this material condenses into chromosomes. The nuclear components communicate with the cytosol via nuclear pores, which are openings in the nuclear envelope.

MITOCHONDRIA

Mitochondria (Greek *mitos* 'thread' + *chondrion*, diminutive of *chondros* 'grain') are responsible for the chemical reactions of respiration. About the same size as bacteria, mitochondria are the power-plants of all eukaryotic cells; they are the sites for ATP synthesis. ATP is the 'energy molecule' of cells. Energy from the breakdown of ATP drives many important cellular reactions. The inner membrane of mitochondria is organised into many inwardly projecting folds known as cristae. It is here that the process of oxidative phosphorylation that generates ATP occurs, while the matrix is where the enzymes of the Krebs cycle and other metabolic pathways are located. Mitochondria are most numerous in cells that use a lot of energy, such as liver and muscle cells.

ENDOPLASMIC RETICULUM

Flattened sheets, sacs, and tubes of membrane extend throughout the cytoplasm of eukaryotic cells, enclosing a large intracellular space. This complex system is called the endoplasmic reticulum (ER) membrane and is in structural continuity with the outer membrane of the nuclear envelope. It specialises in the synthesis and transport of lipids and membrane proteins. The rough endoplasmic reticulum, RER, is the region of the ER associated with ribosomes. RER is involved in the synthesis of secreted and membrane-bound proteins.

The smooth ER is generally more tubular and lacks attached ribosomes. It has a major function in lipid metabolism.

GOLGI APPARATUS

The Golgi apparatus or dictyosome is a system of stacked, membrane-bounded, flattened sacs involved in modifying, sorting, and packing macromolecules for either secretion or delivery to other organelles. The Golgi apparatus is closely related to the endoplasmic reticulum. Around the Golgi apparatus are numerous small membrane-bounded vesicles (50 nm and larger) that carry material between the Golgi apparatus and the different compartments in the cell, or through the cell membrane. The Golgi apparatus is very prominent in secretory cells such as antibody-producing activated plasma cells.

LYSOSOMES

These are the digestive centres of the cell. They are membrane-bounded vesicular organelles formed by the Golgi apparatus, of the order of 0.2–0.5 μm, that contain hydrolytic enzymes involved in intracellular digestions. They allow the cell to digest and thereby remove unwanted substances and structures, especially damaged or foreign structures, such as bacteria.

PEROXISOMES

Peroxisomes are so called because they usually contain one or more enzymes that use molecular oxygen to remove hydrogen atoms from specific organic substrates in an oxidative reaction that produces hydrogen peroxide. They are similar physically to lysosomes in that they are membrane-bounded vesicles of the order of 0.2–0.5 μm. However, they are thought to be formed by budding off from the smooth endoplasmic reticulum rather than the Golgi apparatus, and contain oxidases rather than hydrolases.

CYTOSKELETON

In the cytosol, arrays of protein filaments form networks that give the cell shape and provide a mechanism for movement. The three main kinds of cytoskeletal filaments are microtubules (25 nm diameter), actin filaments (8 nm diameter), and intermediate filaments (10 nm diameter).

The microtubules are involved in controlling the orderly growth of the cell wall and determining the direction of cell expansion, and make up the spindle fibres for dividing cells.

Actin filaments are two-stranded helical polymers of the protein actin. They appear as flexible structures that, although dispersed throughout the cell, are most highly concentrated just beneath the plasma membrane.

The intermediate filaments are rope-like fibres, made of intermediate filament proteins, which constitute a large and heterogeneous family. One type of these filaments forms a meshwork called the nuclear lamina just beneath the inner nuclear membrane. Other types extend across the cytoplasm, providing the cell's mechanical strength and maintaining the mechanical stresses in an epithelial tissue by spanning the cytoplasm from one cell–cell junction to another.

RIBOSOMES

Ribosomes are made up of combinations of RNA and proteins and are the organelles responsible for protein synthesis. These small (~20 nm diameter), spherical structures are the most numerous organelles in almost all cells, and are located in the cytoplasm – either suspended in the cytosol or attached to the surface of the endoplasmic reticulum. Ribosomes are complex organelles that catalyse the synthesis of polypeptides using mRNA templates, by a process known as translation (this will be elaborated later). Eukaryotic ribosomes are larger (80S) than bacterial ribosomes (70S). The differences between the eukaryotic and prokaryotic ribosomes can be exploited in developing novel antibiotics, which kill bacteria by inhibiting only bacterial protein synthesis.

THE GENOME

The thread-like double-helical molecule known as deoxyribonucleic acid (DNA) provides the organism with its identity, referred to as its genome. The DNA is parcelled into genes, which code for proteins, which dictate the inherent properties of a species. The large amount of information that is required by all cells in the body during all the stages of life must be stored, yet be easily accessible, and must be copied reliably during the innumerable cell divisions that take place from conception to cell death. The cells of most plants and animals contain two genomes; such organisms are referred to as diploid. The cells of most fungi, algae, and bacteria contain just one genome; these organisms are called haploid.

The genome itself is made up of extremely long molecules of DNA that are organised into chromosomes. The human body has two sets of 23 chromosomes. Genes are simply the functional regions of chromosomal DNA. Each chromosome in the genome carries a different array of genes. In the diploid cell, each chromosome and the genes within are present twice.

Structure of DNA

Although DNA contains the information necessary for the synthesis of proteins, it does not participate directly in the assembly of protein molecules. Instead, the information contained within DNA must be transferred to ribonucleic acid (RNA) first. This mechanism for expressing genetic information occurs in all living organisms, and has led to what is now called the 'central dogma' of molecular biology: genetic information flows from DNA to RNA and then to protein. In some viruses, genetic information can be transferred from RNA to protein in the absence of DNA, while in other viruses (retroviruses) the flow is from RNA to DNA to RNA to protein. The next section describes in more detail the mechanism by which DNA directs the synthesis of protein.

The genetic code

DNA consists of long strands of sugar residues (deoxyribose) linked together by phosphodiester bonds. As the phosphate moiety links the 3' carbon atom of one sugar to the 5' carbon of the next, the sugar–phosphate backbone is polar: one end of the molecule has a free 3' hydrogen (the 3' end), whereas the other end has a phosphorylated 5' carbon (the 5' end). Attached to each sugar residue is a base, which is either a purine (adenine (A) or guanine (G)) or a pyrimidine (cytosine (C) or thymine (T)). This combination of base and sugar together form a nucleotide, which is the building block of DNA synthesis. In the mature DNA molecule, two of these strands are wound together in an antiparallel fashion (i.e. with one strand running 5' to 3' and the other 3' to 5') to form a double helix (Figure 12.4). Conventionally, when writing the order of bases of a single nucleic acid chain, one begins with the 5' phosphate on the left. In the DNA double helix, the phosphate backbone is on the outside and the bases on the inside.

As described, each nucleotide contains one of four bases, adenine, guanine, cytosine, and thymine (A, G, C, and T). In the double-stranded DNA molecule, bases in one strand are specifically paired, A to T and G to C, with bases in the second strand.

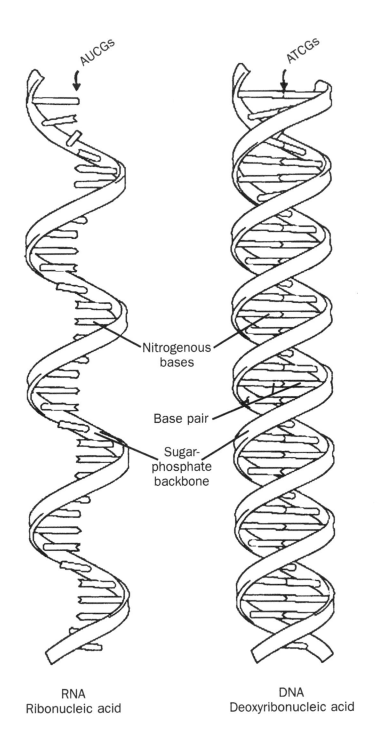

AUCGs

ATCGs

Nitrogenous bases

Base pair

Sugar-phosphate backbone

RNA
Ribonucleic acid

DNA
Deoxyribonucleic acid

Figure 12.4 *Structures of RNA and DNA.*

It is the particular sequence of the nucleotides in a DNA chain that constitutes the blueprint that directs the cellular machinery to synthesise proteins of a particular length and polypeptide sequence. The nucleotide sequences encoding particular amino acids consist of triplets known as codons. Whereas the number of possible codons derived from four bases is 64 ($4 \times 4 \times 4$), only 61 of these combinations code for amino acids; as there are only 20 different amino acids that occur in proteins, more than one codon can code for each amino acid – a feature known as redundancy. Thus, while each codon codes for one amino acid only, each amino acid is encoded by a number of different codons. One particular codon, ATG, which encodes the amino acid methionine, also acts as the START signal from which the cellular machinery will start reading the series of triplet codes encoding a particular protein. The three triplets that do not specify amino acids are known as nonsense codons, these are STOP signals, and cause the termination of polypeptide synthesis.

PROTEIN SYNTHESIS

As protein synthesis occurs on ribosomes, which are located in the cytoplasm and DNA is within the nucleus, a different message must carry genetic information from the nucleus to the cytoplasm. This is achieved by the RNA molecule known as messenger RNA (mRNA). Hence, transfer of genetic information from DNA to protein takes two stages. First, the genetic message is passed from DNA to mRNA (transcription); second, the message in the mRNA passes from the nucleus into the cytoplasm, where it is used to direct the assembly of the specific sequence of amino acids to form a protein (translation) (Figure 12.5).

Transcription: mRNA synthesis

During transcription, the sequence of nucleotides in DNA is used as a template on which to direct the sequence of nucleotides in the mRNA.

The structure of the RNA molecule differs in only a few respects from that of DNA. First, it consists of a single (rather than a double) chain of nucleotides (Figure 12.4). Second, in RNA, the sugar in each nucleotide is ribose rather than deoxyribose. Finally, the pyrimidine base thymine (T) in DNA is replaced in RNA by the pyrimidine base uracil (U), which can base-pair with the purine adenine (A–U pairing, instead of A–T in DNA). The other three bases (adenine, guanine, and cytosine), are the same in both DNA and RNA. The mRNA is synthesised from a pool of free (uncombined) ribonucleotides, each containing three phosphate groups (nucleotide triphosphates): ATP, GTP, CTP, and UTP.

In DNA, the two polynucleotide chains are linked together by hydrogen bonds between specific pairs of bases, A–T and G–C. Transcription starts with the breaking of these hydrogen bonds; hence a portion of the two chains of the DNA double helix separates. The bases in the exposed DNA nucleotides are then able to pair with the bases in the free ribonucleotide triphosphates. Free ribonucleotides containing adenine pair with any exposed thymine base in DNA. Likewise, free ribonucleotides containing G, C, or U pair with the exposed DNA bases C, G, and A, respectively. Thus, the nucleotide sequence in DNA acts as a template that determines the sequence of nucleotides in mRNA.

The aligned ribonucleotides are joined together by the enzyme RNA polymerase. RNA polymerase catalyses the splitting-off of two of the three phosphate groups from each nucleotide and the covalent linkage of the RNA nucleotide to the next one in sequence. The resulting nucleotide sequence in the mRNA is not identical to that in the copied strand of DNA; rather, it is complementary since its formation depends on the pairing between complementary, not identical, bases. Which of the two DNA strands is used as the template for mRNA synthesis is determined by a specific sequence of nucleotides in DNA, called the promoter, located at the beginning of each gene. The promoter, to which RNA polymerase binds, is present in only one of the two DNA strands. Beginning at the promoter end of a gene, the RNA polymerase

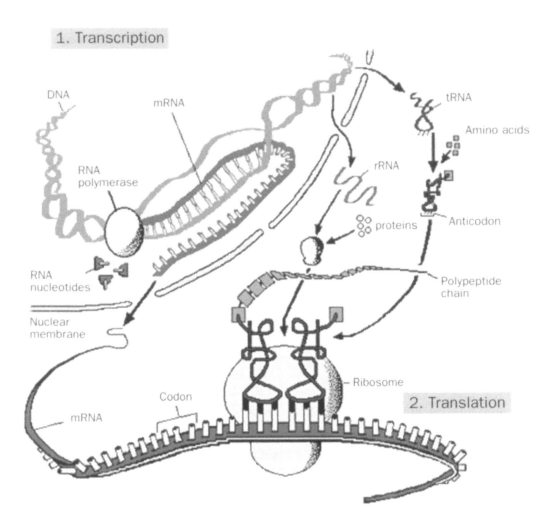

1. Transcription

DNA

mRNA

RNA polymerase

RNA nucleotides

Nuclear membrane

tRNA

Amino acids

rRNA

proteins

Anticodon

Polypeptide chain

Codon

mRNA

Ribosome

2. Translation

Figure 12.5 *Protein synthesis.*

separates the two DNA strands as it moves along one strand, joining one ribonucleotide at a time to the growing mRNA chain until it reaches a termination codon at the end of the gene, and this causes the RNA polymerase to release the newly formed mRNA.

Various mechanisms are used by cells either to block or to make accessible the promoter region of any particular gene. Such regulation of gene transcription provides a means of controlling the synthesis of specific proteins and thereby the activities of the cell.

Although the entire sequence of nucleotides in a gene is transcribed into a corresponding sequence of nucleotides in mRNA, only selected portions of this sequence code for sequences of amino acids; these coding portions are known as exons, the intervening non-coding regions (i.e. those that separate exons) are known as introns.

Before passing into the cytoplasm, a newly formed mRNA must undergo RNA processing to remove the intron sequences. Enzymes that identify nucleotide sequences at the beginning and end of each intron remove the introns and splice the end of one exon to the beginning of another exon to form a contiguous mRNA with no intron segments. Hence the final lengths of the mRNAs are 75–90% shorter than the originally transcribed mRNA. In some cases, the exons derived from a single gene can be spliced together non-sequentially ('alternative splicing'), resulting in the formation of different mRNAs from the same gene and giving rise to several different proteins.

Translation: polypeptide synthesis

Once transcribed and processed, an mRNA molecule will move through the pores in the nuclear envelope into the cytoplasm, where it binds to a ribosome. This is where protein synthesis occurs. Proteins synthesised on free ribosomes are released into the cytosol, whereas those synthesised on bound ribosomes are released into the lumen of the endoplasmic reticulum, from which they are either secreted from the cell or transferred to various organelles.

An essential component of ribosomes is ribosomal RNA (rRNA). The genes that code for rRNA are associated with the nucleolus, which is the site at which the components of ribosome are assembled together.

Each ribosome consists of two subunits: a large 60S and a smaller 40S subunit. When a mRNA molecule arrives in the cytoplasm, one end of it binds to the 40S subunit, and then this combination binds to the 60S subunit to form a fully functional ribosome with a portion of the mRNA lying in a groove between the two subunits. The mRNA is now ready to direct protein assembly. The sequence of codons in mRNA specifies the order of amino acids in the protein, using the triplet code described.

By themselves, free amino acids do not have the ability to bind to the appropriate bases in mRNA codons. This process of identification involves another type of RNA: transfer RNA (tRNA). tRNA molecules are the smallest of the three types of RNA (~80 nucleotides long). The single chain of tRNA loops back upon itself, forming a structure resembling a cloverleaf with three loops. Like the other RNAs, tRNA is encoded by DNA, in this case at specific tRNA genes. tRNA then moves to the cytoplasm. The key to tRNA's role in protein synthesis is that it combines with both a specific amino acid and a

codon in mRNA specific for that amino acid. This permits tRNA to act as the link between an amino acid and the mRNA codon for that amino acid.

The attachment of tRNA to its amino acid is catalysed by the enzyme aminoacyl-tRNA synthetase. There are at least 20 different types of this enzyme, each of which carries out the linkage of a specific amino acid to a particular type of tRNA. The next step is to link the tRNA, bearing its attached amino acid, to the mRNA codon for that amino acid. This is achieved by basepairing between tRNA and mRNA. A threenucleotide sequence at the end of one of the loops of the tRNA can base-pair with the complementary codon in mRNA. This tRNA triplet sequence is appropriately termed an anticodon. Hence the anticodon is a nucleotide triplet in a tRNA molecule that aligns with a particular codon on the mRNA under the influence of the ribosome so that the amino acid carried by the tRNA is ready to be inserted in a growing protein chain.

The individual amino acids linked to mRNA by tRNA must now be linked to each other by the formation of peptide bonds. The ribosome can identify the initial codon sequence in mRNA and will catalyse the formation of a peptide bond between the first and second amino acids in the peptide chain being synthesised. Following the initiation of protein synthesis, the polypeptide chain is elongated by successive addition of amino acids. The 60S subunit has two binding sites for tRNA: one to hold the tRNA that is attached to the most recently added amino acid and the other to hold the tRNA containing the next amino acid to be added to the chain. Ribosomal enzymes catalyse the formation of a peptide bond between these two amino acids. The ribosome will then move forwards so that the next codon and an associated tRNA will occupy one of the binding sites. When the ribosome reaches the termination codon in mRNA specifying the end of the protein, the link between the polypeptide chain and the last tRNA is broken, and the completed protein is released from the ribosome. The same strand of mRNA can be used to synthesise many molecules of the protein because the mRNA molecule is not destroyed during protein assembly. While one ribosome is moving along the strand of mRNA, a second ribosome may become attached to the beginning of the mRNA and begin the synthesis of a second protein molecule. In fact, as many as 70 ribosomes may be attached to the same strand of mRNA at any one time. Eventually, the mRNA is degraded into nucleotides by cytoplasmic enzymes. Thus, unless the gene corresponding to a particular protein continues to be transcribed into mRNA, the synthesis of that protein will eventually slow down and cease as the mRNA is degraded.

Changes can occur in the structure of some polypeptide chains after their synthesis on a ribosome; these changes are collectively known as post-translational modification. For example, certain classes of proteins, known as glycoproteins, are formed by the post-translational addition of various carbohydrate groups to the protein.

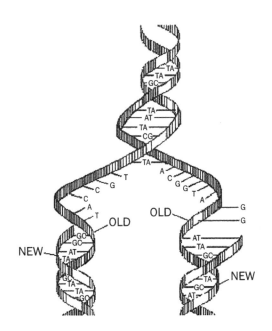

Figure 12.6 *DNA replication.*

DNA replication

The DNA template, via the synthesis of proteins, determines the structure and function of cells. The human body develops from a single cell, the fertilised egg, which must divide many times during embryonic development and growth. Cell division requires the entire DNA genome to be copied (a process known as replication) such that the two resulting daughter cells receive identical copies of the genetic information.

The fundamental property of DNA is that it can duplicate itself without information from any other cellular component – unlike, for example, mRNA which can only be formed in the presence of DNA, or protein, which uses mRNA as a template. Indeed, all other molecules synthesised by a cell are formed by metabolic pathways that are controlled by proteins in the form of enzymes. The replication of DNA follows a similar process to that of mRNA synthesis. During DNA replication, the two strands of the double helix separate, and the exposed bases in each strand base-pair with free deoxyribonucleotide triphosphates (Figure 12.6). The enzyme DNA polymerase then links the free nucleotides together, forming a new strand of DNA. Unlike transcription, during replication,

both strands of the original DNA act as templates for the synthesis of new strands. The end result is two identical double-stranded molecules of DNA. In each copy, there is one strand from the original DNA molecule and one strand that has been newly synthesised. Prior to cell division, the DNA molecules in the nucleus are replicated by this process, and one copy will be passed on to each of the two new cells when the cell divides.

CELL DIVISION

Starting with a single fertilised egg, the first cell division in development produces two cells, which then divide, producing four, and so on. Thus, starting from a single cell, 3 divisions will produce 8 cells (2^3). In fact if the development of the human body involved only the cycle of cell division and growth, it would require only 64 division cycles to produce all the cells in the adult body. This is not the case only because the process of development also involves the programmed death of cells (known as apoptosis). The time between cell divisions varies considerably in different types of cells, with the most rapidly growing cells, such as those in the brush border of the intestinal tract, dividing about once every 24 hours.

The cell cycle is the sets of events that take place during cell division. The cell cycle oscillates between mitosis (M phase) and interphase. Interphase is the cell cycle stage between nuclear divisions, when the DNA in chromosomes is transcriptionally active. DNA replication occurs during interphase about 10 hours prior to the first visible signs of cell division. Since cell division takes about 1 hour, the cell spends most of its time in interphase. Interphase can be subdivided, in order, into G_1 (G stands for 'gap'), S (S for 'synthesis') phase, and G_2. DNA replication takes place during the S phase. The length of the cell cycle is regulated through a special option in G_1 in which G_1 cells can enter a resting phase called G_0. Cell division itself is known as mitosis (Figure 12.7). In cells that give rise to the germ cell (eggs and sperm), the process of cell division is known as meiosis – this differs from mitosis in various ways, particularly in the fact that the cells produced are haploid rather than diploid.

Before cells can divide, the nucleus itself must divide into two daughter nuclei identical with the parent nucleus; following this, the cytoplasm will divide to give two cells (cytokinesis). Although these are two separate events, the term 'mitosis' is often used in a broad sense to include both processes (but actually only truly refers to nuclear division). Mitosis that is not followed by cytokinesis produces the multinucleated cells found in the liver, placenta, among some embryonic cells, and among cancer cells. During most of interphase, DNA is dispersed throughout the nucleus in association with proteins to form extended nucleoprotein threads known as chromatin. Chromatin is the substance of the chromosomes; it includes DNA, chromosomal proteins, and chromosomal RNA. When DNA replicates, each thread of chromatin gives rise to two identical threads known as inter chromatids, which remain paired. As a cell enters mitosis, each chromatid pair becomes highly coiled and condensed, forming the rod-shaped bodies that give rise to our textbook representation of chromosomes (meaning 'coloured bodies', so-called because of their intense staining by the dyes used to visualise structures under a microscope). As the chromosomes condense, the nuclear membrane breaks down, and the chromosomes become linked to spindle fibres, via a specialised region known as the centromere. The spindle fibres, composed of microtubules, generate the forces that divide the cell. The spindle fibres extend between two centrioles located on opposite sides of the cell, which are specialised structures involved in spindle formation and action.

As mitosis proceeds, the sister chromatids in each chromosome separate at the centromere and move toward the opposed centrioles. The spindle fibres act as though they were pulling the chromatids towards the poles, although the actual molecular mechanism of this movement is unclear.

Cytokinesis begins as the sister chromatids separate. The cell begins to constrict along a plane perpendicular to the axis of the mitotic apparatus, and constriction continues until the cell has been pinched in half, forming two daughter cells. Following cytokinesis, the spindle fibres dissolve, a nuclear envelope forms, and the chromatids uncoil in each daughter cell.

CELL DIFFERENTIATION

As identical sets of DNA molecules pass to each of the daughter cells during cell division, every cell in the body, with the exception of the germ cells, contains the same genetic information as every other cell. However, it is possible for one cell to become a muscle cell and synthesise muscle proteins while another cell containing the same genetic information becomes a nerve cell and synthesises a different set of proteins. The formation of different types of cell from a similar precursor is known as differentiation. What underlies differentiation is the fact that different combinations of genes are active in the different cells. The problem of cell differentiation is thus related to the general problem of the regulation of protein synthesis. This regulation can essen-

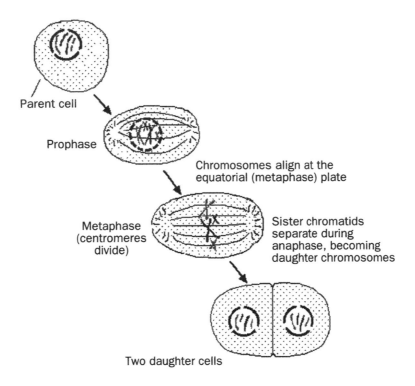

Parent cell

Prophase

Chromosomes align at the
equatorial (metaphase) plate

Metaphase
(centromeres
divide)

Sister chromatids
separate during
anaphase, becoming
daughter chromosomes

Two daughter cells

Figure 12.7 *Mitosis.*

tially be effected at four steps in the process that leads from DNA to the final protein:

1. Regulation of gene transcription into mRNA can alter the rate of mRNA formation.
2. Regulation of mRNA processing can produce different combinations of exons or alter the ability of mRNA to associate with a ribosome.
3. Regulation of the stability of processed mRNA – the length of time the mRNA stays in the cytoplasm before it is broken down – can control the number of protein molecules formed from a molecule of mRNA.
4. Regulation of mRNA translation can alter the rate at which a protein is assembled on a ribosome.

Beyond each of these, the cell can also regulate the *activity* of the completed protein by allosteric and covalent modifications. The most important level of regulation is that of gene transcription, i.e. certain genes are 'turned on' or 'turned off'

in different cell types, resulting in a different profile of proteins being present. A great deal is known about the signals that control the transcription of specific genes. The transcription of individual genes is switched on and off in cells by gene regulatory proteins. Gene regulatory proteins recognise specific DNA sequences and thereby determine which of the thousands of genes in a cell will be transcribed. In prokaryotes, these proteins usually bind to specific DNA sequences close to the RNA polymerase start site and (depending on the nature of the regulatory protein and the precise location of its binding site relative to the start site) either activate or repress transcription of genes. Although prokaryotic RNA polymerases can initiate transcription on there own, eukaryotic polymerases require the prior assembly of general transcription factors at the promoter. These general transcription factors are part of the mechanism of transcription as distinct from its regulation. In eukaryotes, gene transcription is generally controlled by combinations of gene regulatory proteins. It is thought that each type of cell in a higher eukaryotic organism contains a specific combination of gene regulatory proteins that ensures the expression of only those genes appropriate to that type of cell. A given gene regulatory protein may be expressed in a variety of circumstances, and typically is involved in the regulation of many genes.

During embryonic development, cells must differentiate in a specific spatial and temporal order. Although much is still to be learnt about the control of this process, it is clear that communication between cells is essential. The pathways by which cells respond to an external stimulus are collectively known as signal transduction; examples of these processes will be described in the next section.

SIGNAL TRANSDUCTION

Signal transduction consists of a series of events that allow a signal received by a transmembrane receptor to have a functional consequence within the cell. This signal may be a small molecule such as a hormone or a cytokine or it may be a component of the extracellular matrix or indeed a molecule attached to an adjacent cell.

The combination of such a signal (or messenger) with a receptor causes a change in the conformation of the receptor known as receptor activation. This is the initial response in signal transduction, which can lead to:

- changes in the cell's membrane permeability, in the rates at which it transports various substances, or its electrical state;
- changes in the rate at which a particular substance is synthesised or secreted by the cell;
- changes in the strength of contraction, if the cell is a muscle cell.

Despite the seeming variety of these ultimate responses, there is a common denominator. They are all due directly to alterations of particular cellular proteins, which is the end result of signal transduction.

The receptors involved in signal transduction can act in various ways. The receptor when activated may open or close a membrane ion channel, resulting in an electrical signal or changes in, for instance, calcium concentrations. Ca^{2+} then acts as a so-called second messenger, which serves as a relay from the plasma membrane to the biochemical machinery within the cells. The calcium ion is one of the most widespread second messengers, and an activated receptor can increase cytosolic calcium in several ways:

- It can open membrane calcium channels, hence allowing the influx of extracellular calcium.
- It may activate the membrane enzyme phospholipase C, which breaks down phosphatidylinositol bisphosphate (PIP_2) to inositol trisphosphate (IP_3) and diacylglycerol (DAG). IP_3 stimulates the release of calcium from the endoplasmic reticulum.

Calcium binds to one of several intracellular proteins, most often calmodulin. Calcium-activated calmodulin activates or inhibits many proteins, including calmodulin-dependent protein kinases. Protein kinases are enzymes that phosphorylate other proteins by transferring to them a phosphate group from ATP. This introduction of the phosphate group is a post-translational modification (referred to above) that changes the activity of the protein, often itself an enzyme. Because DAG itself can activate protein kinase C (which phosphorylates many protein substrates), a single messenger may recruit multiple pathways, each of which may trigger a different response.

Alternatively, receptors may interact with a G protein. G proteins (so-called because they bind to guanosine triphosphate (GTP) with high affinity) are a family of plasma membrane-bound regulatory proteins with which many activated receptors interact and ultimately alter. The altered G protein then interacts with another protein – either an ion channel or an enzyme – in the plasma membrane to elicit the next step in the sequence of events leading to the cell's response. The G protein consists of three subunits, α, β, and γ, of molecular weights 42, 35, and 10 kDa respectively. G proteins are not second messengers themselves as they do not pass information directly from the plasma membrane into the cell, although they do contribute to the generation of second messengers. Some G proteins result in the activation or inhibition of the membrane enzyme adenylate cyclase, which catalyses the conversion of ATP to cyclic adenosine monophosphate (cAMP). cAMP then acts as a second messenger to activate intracellular cAMP-dependent protein kinase. This protein kinase phosphorylates proteins that mediate the cell's ultimate response to the first message. Cyclic guanosine monophosphate (cGMP), formed by the action of membrane guanylate cyclases, also functions as a second messenger through a protein kinase.

This type of cascade is an extremely efficient system for amplifying the signal, since the binding of an agonist (e.g. adrenaline) molecule results in the activation of adenylate cyclase molecules, and the generation of many molecules of cAMP.

Each cell in a multicellular animal is programmed during development to respond to a specific set of signals that act in various combinations to regulate the behaviour of the cell and to determine whether the cell lives or dies and whether it proliferates or stays quiescent. Most of these signals are known as paracrine, in which local mediators are rapidly taken up, destroyed, or immobilised, so that they act only on neighbouring cells. In addition, centralised control is exerted by endocrine signalling, in which circulating hormones target cells throughout the body, and by synaptic signalling, in which neurotransmitters secreted by nerve cells act locally on the postsynaptic cells that their axons contact.

Cell signalling requires both extracellular signalling molecules and a complementary set of membrane receptor proteins in each cell that enable it to bind and respond to them in a programmed and characteristic way. Some small hydrophobic signalling molecules, including the steroid and thyroid hormones and the retinoids, are actually able to diffuse across the plasma membrane of the target cell and then interact with intracellular receptor proteins, which directly regulate the transcription of specific genes.

Embryonic cells must not only become different; they must also remain different even after the influence that initiated cell diversification has disappeared. This requires cell memory, which enables cells to become determined for a particular specialised role long before they differentiate overtly. The mechanisms of cell memory may be cytoplasmic, involving molecules in the cytoplasm that act back on the nucleus to maintain their own synthesis, autocrine, involving secreted molecules that act back on the cell, or nuclear, involving processes of chromatin or DNA modification. In some cases, the state of determination has been related to the expression of specific regulatory genes, such as the myogenic genes for muscle cells.

The different kinds of cells in an embryo are produced in a regular spatial pattern. The formation of this pattern usually begins with asymmetries in the egg and continues by means of cell–cell interactions in the embryo. The spatial signals that coordinate pattern formation supply cells with positional information, and a cell's remembered record of this information is called its positional value. Cells in the early forelimb and hindlimb rudiments of a vertebrate embryo, for example, acquire different positional values, making forelimb and hindlimb cells non-equivalent in their intrinsic character, long before the detailed pattern of cell differentiation has been determined.

In many animals, the pattern of positional values is closely coupled to the control of cell proliferation according to a simple rule of intercalation. According to this rule, discontinuities of positional value provoke local cell proliferation, and the newly formed cells take on intermediate positional values that restore continuity in the pattern. This mechanism is likely to operate in normal embryonic development to correct inaccuracies in the initial specification of positional information.

FURTHER READING

Alberts B, Bray D, Lewis J, et al. *Molecular Biology of the Cell*, 4th edn. London: Garland, 2001.

Bullock, Boyle, Wang. *NMS Physiology*. Philadelphia: Williams & Wilkins.

Guyton. *Textbook of Medical Physiology*. Philadelphia: WB Saunders.

Lowery, Siekevitz, Menniger, Gallant. *Cell Structure and Function: An Integrated Approach*. Philadelphia: Saunders College.

Index